How to Have

RADIANT
HEALTH

Joy Haney

Radiant Life Publications
Stockton, CA

How to Have
RADIANT HEALTH

Contents:

Acknowledgments

Special thanks to the following people who helped make this book possible:

Pamela L.Byrne, Ph.D., R.N., who gave me excellent advice and who authored the foreword.

Siri Khalsa, health counselor, who allowed me to use material from her monthly publication, "Nutrition News."

Mary Kloepper, wife of Dr. Kloepper, who supported and encouraged me.

Elizabeth Shivers, my capable secretary and one of the proof-readers.

Bill Riddell, who gave of his time and excellent computer skills.

Joanie McCulloch, who works at Artesian Health Store, and has so cheerfully and willingly secured needed information for me from time to time.

Kenneth Haney, my husband, who encourages me to write and is patient and understanding during my times of inspiration and meeting deadlines.

What readers have said:

"A must have, Gem of a book, for anyone seeking answers for obtaining, keeping, or regaining health. Well written, informative information. Truly useful!"

Dr. Lynn Hill N.D.
Cleveland, GA

"I have read a great number of health books, but yours is so concise and full of good health practices, that I have to say it rates right up there on top. I bought a copy for the nurse in my mother's doctor's office. She thanked me for the wonderful informative book, and said she found it to be of great value to her family."

Grace Jorgensen
Racine, WI

"Regarding the book on good health, I had changed my cooking and eating habits some time ago, but knew I didn't have the 'big picture.' *Radiant Health* is so full of documented, researched information, written in layman's terms, and anointed by the Holy Spirit; well, there is just no comparison."

Alice Tanner
Stockton, CA

Foreword

How to Have Radiant Health is a collection of concise, informative and inspirational ideas on health and wellness. Presentation of this book could not be more timely as the nature of health care in the United States is changing. The "sick-role model," where individuals have relied on the medical establishment for complete care, is evolving into a "self-management and/or partnership with the provider" model. Partnering with the provider and self-management encourages a greater degree of individual responsibility for health and control of risk factors. The ability to demonstrate control is an important factor in health. The World Health Organization (WHO) has incorporated this into its current definition of health: a process of enabling individuals and communities to increase control over the determinants of health. Control is used not in the sense of manipulating oneself or others, rather in the context of influencing the course of one's life through the use of individual choice. Central to the process of self-management is health knowledge, healthy lifestyle choice (control of risk factors) and preventive maintenance behaviors.

Behavioral and Preventive Medicine research clearly demonstrate the benefits of positive health choice and control of risk factors, a few examples are the following: stress management techniques have the potential to decrease hypertension, headaches, pain, and anxiety, a healthful low-fat diet may reduce cholesterol, cardiac vessel disease, obesity, gastrointestinal symptoms, and exercise or stretching activities may decrease hypertension, isolation, and improve function, flexibility and mood.

My professional experience in the field of health care, research on health activity and personal dedication to mind-body wellness for over twenty years, vigorously supports the demonstrated effectiveness of positive health choice and control of lifestyle risk factors. Patients have taught me that a reduction of risk factors, attitudinal enhancement, relaxation techniques, healthful diet, exercise/stretching habits, positive recreational choices, clarification of one's life purpose, relationship connections, spiritual awareness, contribute to optimal health and wellness.

I am enthusiastic about *Radiant Health* and believe it can change lives. It provides a unifying framework for the development of positive health and wellness. Personal health responsibility (choice and control) is highlighted while practical information about universal laws of health and relationships is provided. New choice options (self-management) point the way to greater vitality, harmony, and happiness. In the widest sense, *Radiant Health* is a guide to joyous, balanced-healthful living and given the mounting evidence–often from disparate fields such as philosophy, biology, medicine, pharmacology, nutrition, psychology, education, business, and religion–which describes the restorative power of inner peace and love, the collective benefits of this book are unlimited . . . .

Pamela L. Byrne, Ph.D., RN
Health Psychologist-Registered nurse
Coordinator of Behavioral Health,
Coordinator of Chronic Pain Management & Prevention Service
Kaiser Permanente

Preface

Why am I writing this book? Let me go back to the year 1974. December 18, 1974, my mother died with cancer of the cervix. Prior to this, my father, mother, and ten-year-old sister lived with my husband and I, and our four children for approximately six months. During that time I bathed mother, took care of her, and watched her die. Even though it was a stressful time, it was probably one of the most precious times of my life, being with her in those few, short months.

With the extra care of my mother (I also had four children ages 4-11 at that time), I experienced great physical distress for three months after the funeral. Because I was experiencing chest pains and suffering with high blood pressure, my husband took me to the doctor three different times where they did EKG tests. Finally, the doctor told me I was suffering from severe stress, exhaustion, and grief.

Upon the doctor's advice my husband took me to a small mountain town called Sonora, in the state of California, for two days to rest and relax. Little did I know, but that trip was to change my whole life in the field of health and nutrition. As we were walking down the street, I noticed a health store, which was rather a new thing back then, and so we decided to go inside. The book that drew my attention was entitled something like, *How to be Healthy and Live to Be A Hundred Years Old.* We bought the book, (sorry to say, it has been misplaced), but it opened a whole new world to me.

I began to study and research the subject of health and nutrition, and since then have taught on this subject at a local college and at different seminars. I do not claim to be an expert, just an enlightened reader. I know that it works because it has helped me, my family, and a host of friends and other people. I believe that the information presented in this book should be available to the public.

This book will join many other books that speak to the public about their health and general well-being. It does not take away from physicians or registered dietitians, but adds food for thought, and some tried and true remedies and "suggestions" that have worked for us and others.

Author's note: *The medical information and procedures contained in this book are not intended as a substitute for consulting, and/or being under the care of your physician. Any attempt to diagnose and treat an illness should come under the direction of a physician who is familiar with nutrition therapy.*

Because there is always some risk involved when dealing with serious illnesses, the author and publisher are not responsible for any adverse consequences resulting from the use of any of the suggestions in this book. All matters regarding your physical health should be supervised by a medical professional.

Introduction

"He hath made everything beautiful" (Ecclesiastes 3:11). From the beginning God made all things perfect and beautiful; but along with His creation He also instituted laws. When the laws are broken the results are disastrous.

The Earth and Universe are ruled by laws and regulations. Man is also given laws, both physical and spiritual laws, which help guide him to physical and spiritual health. If health laws are broken, or tampered with, whether by accident or intentionally, man's body will suffer.

We have heard that "beauty is in the eye of the beholder," but everyone will agree that radiant health is beautiful. There is something satisfying and inspiring to see vigorous, glowing health in people whether they be 12 or 80. A person that enjoys continual health for the most part is probably obeying most of the laws of physical and mental health.

This book will introduce you to more healthful living, and lead you into making choices that will help you feel better and look better. You will choose whether you live in total health or whether you will seek to have some kind of healthful lifestyle.

Gayelord Hauser, noted health expert, says, "Age is a physiological and psychological matter. Examination of men and women over one hundred years of age at some of our famous clinics revealed that they had four outstanding qualities:

Strong digestive juices
Slow rhythmic heartbeat
Good elimination
Happy dispositions" [1]

Food, vitamins, minerals, and other subjects discussed in this book have something to do with all four things.

Special Note: The information in this book is for educational purposes only and is not intended to replace proper medical care, to diagnose or to prescribe. Proper medical attention should not be avoided, discarded or delayed when there is a reason to seek professional help. However, as soon as you begin or engage in the practice of a healthy lifestyle, most likely you may notice a reduction in the need for medical attention. This is called *preventive medicine.*

The following rules of health were taken from *Poor Richard's Almanack,* 1743, written by Benjamin Franklin, and are quite sensible.

Eat and drink such an exact quantity as the constitution of thy body allows of, in reference to the services of the mind.

They that study much ought not to eat as much as those that work hard.

Excess in all other things whatever, as well as in meat and drink, is also to be avoided.

Youth, age, and sick require a different quantity.

And so do those of contrary complexions; for that which is too much for a phlegmatic man, is not sufficient for a choleric.

The measure of food ought to be (as much as possibly may be) exactly proportionable to the quality and condition of the stomach, because the stomach digests it.

That quantity that is sufficient, the stomach can perfectly concoct and digest, and it sufficeth the due nourishment of the body.

A greater quantity of some things may be eaten than of others, some being of lighter digestion than others.

The difficulty lies in finding out an exact measure; but eat for necessity, not pleasure for lust knows not where necessity ends.

Wouldst thou enjoy a long life, a healthy body, and a vigorous mind, and be acquainted also with the wonderful works of God, labor in the first place to bring thy appetite to reason.

It was Thomas Edison that said, "The doctor of the future will give no medicine, but will interest his patient in the care of the human frame, in diet and in the cause and prevention of disease." Whether Thomas Edison proves to be right, remains unseen for now, but there is a growing interest among patients and doctors in preventing disease by taking proper care of the body and mind. May the information contained in these pages help to enlighten your understanding, and may you enjoy *radiant health* all the days of your life.

Chapter 1

Wonderfully and Fearfully Made

King David of ancient days wrote in Psalm 139:14, "I will praise thee; for I am fearfully and wonderfully made."

The *World Encyclopedia* gives the following information about the human body: "The human body is made up mostly of billions of *cells* so small they can be seen only with a microscope. One drop of blood no bigger than this letter *a* contains 5,000,000 red blood cells and about 5,000 white blood cells. Some cells of the body manufacture and maintain the material that forms bone and cartilage. Different types of cells group together to form various kinds of *tissues*. The tissues in turn form such *organs* as the heart, lungs, and stomach. Organs work together in various *systems* to keep the body running.

"The cells of the body contain water, proteins, fats, sugars, and starch. These substances mainly contain hydrogen, oxygen, and carbon. Proteins contain nitrogen in addition to hydrogen, oxygen, and carbon. The cells have small amounts of certain mineral salts, vitamins, and enzymes. Some cells contain large amounts of certain chemicals."

Some interesting facts about the body are as follows:

The Heart: "The heart beats an average of 75 times a minute, forty million times a year, or two and a half billion times in a life of 70 years. At each beat, the average adult heart discharges about four ounces of blood. This amounts to three thousand gallons a day or 650,000 gallons a year (enough to fill more than 81 tank cars of 8,000 gallons each).

"The heart does enough work in one hour to lift a 150-pound man to the top of a three-story building, enough energy in twelve hours to lift a 65-ton tank car one foot off the ground, or enough power in seventy years to lift the largest battleship afloat completely out of the water." [1]

Cells: "There are several trillion hard-working cells in every person. A cell is so small it takes 250 of them, placed side by side, to equal the diameter of a dot. Inside the membrane of each cell, swimming around in the cytoplasm, are about 200 of these wiggling, squirming particles, each one a living and active chemical laboratory, a food and energy factory.

"Inside of each of these cells are about 200 wiggling mitochondria. Each one of these would be about 1/50,000th the size of a globe as big as a dot! Inside of each mitochondrion are hundreds of small 'spheres' scattered along stalks in the mitochondrion. Each sphere is about 1/1,000th the size of the mitochondrion! So, each sphere would be about one-five-millionth (1/5000,000) the size of a dot! Each of these tiny spheres is a chemical factory, with a 'production line' that produce energy and food for the cell. This is such a marvel of smallness and intricate complexity that it stretches one's imagination even to try to think of it." [2]

Eyes: "No scientific instrument is as sensitive to the light as a person's eye. And in the dark, its sensitivity increases 100,000 times; one can detect a faint glow, less than a thousandth as bright as a candle's flame. He can see light from the stars, and the nearest of all stars is 25 billion miles away.

"Automatically, the muscles of the eye relax so that the lens is small and thick for distant viewing or they stretch the lens to bring into focus. No wonder the eye was the original model for cameras.

Ears: "The ear is as much an acoustic marvel as the eye is an optic one. The inner ear is like a keyboard with 15,000 keys, because that is the number of different tones that can be detected. Not only does the ear perform the function of hearing, it acts to control equilibrium as well. Who but God could have originated such a dual purpose instrument?[3]

Brain: The brain is capable of storing as much as 10 times more information than there is in the library of Congress, with its 17 million volumes.

"Scientists were asked to determine the size, the cooling system, and the power required to perform electronically the same functions that are automatically accomplished by a man's brain during his lifetime. They decided that if all parts were transistorized and built on a miniature scale like those used in rockets to the moon, the following would be needed: A machine the size of the United Nations building in New York; a cooling system with an output equal to Niagara Falls; and a power source that would produce as much electricity as is used in homes, industries, and factories in the entire state of California." [4]

The human body is the most amazing creation on the earth today. Nothing can compare with the intricate workings of the inner and outer man. Only God could create such a wonder. In many cases, He made the body to heal itself if the proper nutrients are present, as well as other factors, which will be discussed in this book.

Chapter 2

Above All: Prosper and Be in Health!

John the Beloved, wrote in III John: 2, "Beloved, I wish above all things thou mayest prosper and be in health, even as thy soul prospereth."

Health means more than not being sick. It gives you a feeling of good spirit. When you are healthy you say you "feel great." You are happier and do better in your work. Health helps you enjoy what you are doing, and as a whole includes physical, mental, spiritual and social health.

Gayla Foster, a friend who lives in Texas, related to me about a time in her life when she felt awful and was quite sick. After going to the doctor and running many tests, he finally told her, "I have good news and bad news, Gayla. The good news is that what you have is not as serious as what we thought it was (cancer). (She was diagnosed with

Chronic Urethritis, which is an inflammation of the urethra. The pain is similar to a severe bladder infection, or cystitis.) The bad news is that there is no cure; it is a chronic illness and, as you know, very painful." She asked, "You mean to tell me I've got to live like this the rest of my life?" He just looked at her and said, "I'm sorry. I know how you feel because I have the same thing. If I could do anything for it, I would have already cured myself. You're just going to have to live with it the rest of your life."

She says she clearly remembers walking out of his office wanting to slam the door off its hinges, but she didn't because she was too ill. She said to herself, "I will not live like this. I will not accept this!" So began her long journey on the road to good health.

She said she learned that her lifestyle and eating habits had everything to do with this particular illness. She wrote to me, "My diet was typical southern: foods rich in animal proteins, e.g., fats from hogs and beef, etc. Accompanying these meats were biscuits and breads (made from white flour), white rice, mashed or fried potatoes, and sugary desserts. Just the combination of these foods is enough to make one very sick within time."

She continues, "The doctor never once told me anything about a change of diet. But he did tell me that I would need to continue having my urethra dilated. I later found out that over a period of time this procedure causes scar tissue and brings about other complications. Surgery at this point was not suggested. However, he prescribed sedatives to relieve the pain and antibiotics to fight the infection and fever.

"It was at this point that I found a licensed nutritionist who then introduced me to the Reams Diet, of MPA. This was fifteen years ago . . . I did find a better way: a nutritional lifestyle!"

I received this letter on January 15, 1995, and she told me she was totally healed and feels wonderful. She is on no medication; she only had a change of diet, iniated an exercise program three times a week, and takes every known vitamin, mineral, and other health giving supplements. In looking over her diet, I noticed it is rich in fresh vegetables, fruits, whole-grains, lean meats and fish, natural seasonings, honey instead of sugar, and based on the adage, "Don't live to eat, but eat to live."

Life should be lived abundantly, but it is difficult to live abundantly when you feel sick. Natural foods are gifts from God, and often we turn our noses up at them, choosing a surgary sweet instead of God's sweet apple. So when the body becomes overloaded with white sugar and white flour, it often responds with headaches, sluggishness, poor skin tone, and vague pains, etc.

The key is developing a lifestyle of healthful choices based on vitamin and mineral content in the food. There are many things that are necessary for good health, but the six basic ingredients that the body cannot do without are vitamins, minerals, fats, carbohydrates, protein and water.

It is important to start living a healthful lifestyle as soon as possible, instead of waiting until one is older and then try to repair the damage done through years of neglect and abuse. Gershon Lesser, MD, says in his book, *Growing Younger: Nutritional Rejuvenation for People Over Forty,* "Those foods highest in nutrients are the best fuel for our bodies."

Roy L. Walford, MD, one of the country's leading authorities on aging and a UCLA pathology professor, wrote in his book, *The 120-Year Diet,* that the life span could be extended through diet. Dr. Walford lists some of the anti-aging super foods as being: black Chinese mushrooms, broccoli, Brussels sprouts, cabbage, carrots, cauliflower, garlic, ginger, lentils, oat bran, onions, parsley, peaches, red pepper, scallions, spinach, sweet potatoes, and whole grains.

Robin Mather wrote an interesting article called *Chicken Soup,* in the Stockton Record, February 8, 1995. She says, "In every culture where chicken is eaten, chicken soup is credited with near magical restorative powers. Put a lot of garlic in and hot chiles; stir in ginger, to…One doctor calls such soup 'the best cold remedy there is.'…Capsaicin, the compound that makes chile peppers hot, has a chemical similarity to guaifenesin, the expectorant found in about 75 over-the-counter and prescription cough syrups, including Robitussin, Vicks Formula 44D and Sudafed. Expectorants loosen chest congestion, which makes it easier to cough up what's clogging your lungs"

Mrs. Mather continues to write, "'A lot of over-the-counter drugs for colds and coughs and bronchitis do exactly what peppers do, but I believe more in peppers.' Dr. Irwin Ziment, a lung specialist at UCLA, has written, 'Peppers don't cause any side effects. I am convinced that 90 percent of all people can tolerate hot food and get a benefit.'"

She gives interesting information about an amino acid found in chicken. "'Chicken, like most protein foods, contains a natural amino acid called cysteine, which is released when you make the soup. Cysteine bears a remarkable chemical similarity to a drug called acetylcysteine, which doctors prescribe for their patients with bronchitis and respiratory infections.'"

Although good foods are important, there are other things that are conducive to good health also. The 12 basic rules for good health are the following things:

- Eat a healthy balanced diet.
- Exercise regularly.
- Get enough sleep. Sleep lets the body rid itself of poison, repair tissues, and grow properly.
- Get enough fresh air and oxygen. Although there is continuous oxygen in all environments, (some rooms/environments may contain toxic allergens which are unhealthy for us); therefore, fresh clean

unpolluted air as well as sunshine is nourishing and valuable.
- Take care of your teeth. Germs form from decayed teeth and may also spread bacteria throughout the body.
- Keep clean. (personal hygiene and living area)
- Dress comfortably–no constricting clothing or shoes.
- Enjoy your work.
- Think healthy thoughts.
- Relax regularly.
- Help others.
- Take vitamins, minerals, and other healthy supplements.

There are certain laws which govern the consistency of the cycle of the earth. Every area of life operates according to set laws by the Creator. The field of physiology, hygiene, botany, zoology, astronomy are all governed by laws. There are civil laws, moral laws, dietary laws, judicial laws; everything is run by precision and established standards.

In Old Testament Bible days, there were certain fowls, animals and fish that could be eaten (namely fowls with the gizzard that separates and cleanses all matter before it becomes flesh, animals that had a divided hoof, and fish which had fins and scales), and some that could not be; these were considered scavengers or unclean animals. Why did

God make these type of fowls, animals and fish? They will eat dead and filthy things, which keeps disease from spreading over the earth and keep the ocean and rivers clean.

Since the body you have been given is a gift from your Creator, it should be treated with respect and attention should be given to the foods that are allowed to be consumed by it. Some people become so used to feeling sluggish, slightly depressed, or experiencing an occasional headache, or dull pain in different parts of the body, that they feel this is normal. It is normal, for those that treat their bodies as if they were made of steel, and as if nothing could harm them.

What is wrong about being selective about what you eat, if you have the privilege of being selective? If you had the choice of choosing between a Lexus automobile or a run-down rattletrap of a car, which would you choose? It is the same way with foods; some are of the Lexus quality, others are in the class of the rattletrap. The rattletrap may finally get you where you are going, (or it may not get you there at all), and if it does, you probably will have a few costly breakdowns along the way, some exasperation, and desperate vows that you will try to get a better car next time.

The only difference is, you can trade a car in for a new one, but you cannot trade your body in for a new one. You can begin today by helping to change the damage that has been done, or to enhance a lifestyle that has already been started toward good nutritional understanding, because the inner workings of the body rebuilds itself every seven years. How it rebuilds will be enhanced by what you have fed into it consistently. There are many variables which affect new cell patterns and growth.

Chapter 3

Vitamins, the Spark Plugs

Gayelord Hauser, author and health counselor, compares the body to a motor car. He says vitamins and minerals are its spark plugs and are essential to the utilization of food and its assimilation into the blood stream. Vitamins are also powerful chemical "regulators." They stimulate growth and regulate body activities.

"Every day millions of cells in your body become worn out, damaged, or destroyed. Every day your body is trying to replace, rebuild, and repair these cells in order to maintain your health and prevent illness. But in order to accomplish this gigantic task it must have sufficient and effective repair materials. The only way your body can get these repair materials is from your diet. There is no other way." [1]

Vitamins together with minerals help to ignite the use of the body's fuel. Linda Clark tells a true story about a horse. Some neighbors were moving away and had agreed to sell their somewhat elderly mare to another neighbor who had two small children. Several months later the original owners returned to visit the horse and were shocked at her appearance. "She looks awful," they said, "Call the vet, quickly."

When they called the vet, he asked several questions, one of them being, "Do you give her vitamins?" The neighbor was surprised and said, "No, am I supposed to?"

"If you want a beautiful, frisky animal, you do," he answered.

"So he outlined a diet. It was to include certain amounts of alfalfa (a whole, natural food); oats (another whole, natural, high-protein food); and in case some of the necessary repair material might be missing from these foods, he added a third natural product which included a combination of many grains, proteins, minerals, and vitamins. On top of all that he prescribed daily, 4 ounces of vitamin-mineral supplement.

"In two weeks you would not have recognized that horse! Her dull coat had become shiny. She held up her once droopy head. The children exclaimed, "Before, we couldn't get her to move fast at all. Now she wants to trot and gallop." [2]

Vitamins are found in food, but due to several modern reasons, the body needs vitamin supplements. According to Dr. Daniel T. Quigley, author of the *The National Malnutrition,* "Everyone who has in the past eaten processed sugar, white flour, or canned food has some deficiency disease, the extent of the disease depending on the percentage of such deficient food in the diet."

Because many restaurants tend to reheat food or keep it warm under heat lamps, if you eat out often, you run the possibility of the risk of vitamin A, B1, and C deficiencies. Many foods today have been processed and depleted in nutrients. Dr. Earl Mindell, author of *The Vitamin Bible,* says that many breads and cereals are high in nothing but carbohydrates, and when they say enriched, it usually means that they have taken out twenty-two natural nutrients and replaced it with only three B vitamins, vitamin D, calcium and iron salts.

Note: A vitamin supplement is no substitute for food, and neither can vitamins be assimilated without ingesting food.

All vitamins are important, but one I would like to bring to your attention especially is Vitamin C. Humans do not produce Vitamin C in their body; therefore it must be taken orally. From the book, *The Vitamin C Connection,* authored by Cheraskin, Ringsdorf, and Sisley, comes the following quote.

"What this country needs is a good five cent pill–some 'magic,' easy-to-swallow little pellet that can slow aging, minimize heart disease, aid recovery from dozens of infectious and degenerative ailments, and inoculate us against countless health problems that stem from emotional stress and environmental pollutants."

In their book the authors explain that we have that "magic" pellet in Vitamin C. To again quote *The Vitamin C Connection:* "Vitamin C is unique among all vitamins. It serves as a kind of special *glue* that holds cells together. Thus, it plays a role in every tissue and organ in the body. A deficiency contributes more damage to more places in the body and creates more biochemical chaos than any other single nutrient."

We learn from Dr. Robert Cathcart's book, *Vitamin C, Titrating to Bowel Tolerance,* that he has personally treated over 9,000 patients with megadoses of Vitamin C. His work shows that persons who have sufficient amounts of C in their bodies to help them withstand severe stress, can expect to overcome the major health problems that would ordinarily be a result of ascorbate insufficiency.

The importance of vitamin C to the stress response cannot be overemphasized. All disease and illness cause stress, surgery and any kind of injury cause stress, and allergic reactions cause stress. Emotional reactions, good or bad, cause stress.

Stress response is based on adrenal response and adrenal response is based on the availability of vitamin C. The need for vitamin C increases with the level of the stress impact.

Stress causes the release of histamine into the bloodstream. Histamine reactions are famous companions of colds, allergy reactions, hayfever and asthma. Vitamin C has antihistamine action, and destroys the histamine molecule. Histamines actually stymie the flow of air in and out of the lungs, whereas Vitamin C brings relief from this kind of air flow restriction.

' Mental stress has as much need for Vitamin C as does physical stress, and it improves people's sense of well-being, seeming to work against anxiety, tension, pain, and other stresses.

People who are on medication, women using the pill, people using aspirin, all need extra amounts of Vitamin C. The granulated form of ascorbic acid was first introduced into our home several years ago by a close friend. Since then we have tried never to be without it. It is my practice to take between 1/2 to 1 teaspoon a day mixed in a small amount of juice. This is between 3,000-5,000 milligrams a day. If any one in the family feels a sore throat coming on, immediately they start taking 1/2 teaspoon of ascorbic acid several times throughout the day. It knocks it everytime.

Adelle Davis was one of the country's best known nutritionists, who studied at Purdue

University, graduated from the University of California at Berkeley, and took postgraduate work at Columbia University and the University of California at Los Angeles before receiving her Master of Science degree in biochemistry from the University of Southern California Medical School. She has authored several books and her book, *Let's Eat Right to Keep Fit*, published in 1970 is still referred to by nutritionists today.

She tells about Dr. Fred R. Klenner, who was chief of staff at the Memorial Hospital in Reidsville, North Carolina, who also authored the book, *The Use of Vitamin C as an Antibiotic*. It is interesting to note that he administered large doses of Vitamin C through injections to patients who were too ill to swallow it. She tells how she visited him and attended one of his lectures. She writes, "He showed slides of hospital records and fever charts and told of case after case of meningitis, encephalitis, virus pneumonia, and serious complications following scarlet fever and other diseases treated with massive amounts of vitamin C. Many patients had not been expected to live; often huge amounts of antibiotics had been given without success; in most cases, fevers ranged from 103 degree to 105 degrees. Within a few minutes after the vitamin was injected, fevers started to drop and temperatures frequently reached normal within a few hours... The initial dose was 2,000 to 6,000 milligrams (2 to 6 grams), followed four and eight hours later by a second and third injection of

2,000 to 4,000 milligrams if the temperature did not remain normal; injections were continued around the clock when needed.

"Dr. Klenner told of an eighteen-month-old girl suffering from polio. The mother reported that the child had become paralyzed following a convulsion, after which she soon lost consciousness. When Dr. Klenner first saw the child, her little body was blue and cold to the touch; he could neither hear heart sounds nor feel her pulse... The only sign of life he could detect was a suggestion of moisture condensed on a mirror held to her mouth... Dr. Klenner injected 6,000 milligrams of vitamin C into her blood; four hours later the child was cheerful and alert, holding a bottle with her right hand, though her left side was paralyzed. A second injection was given; soon the child was laughing and holding her bottle with both hands, all signs of paralysis gone. Dr. Klenner quite understandably speaks of vitamin C as 'the antibiotic par excellence.' A physician who later obtained striking results at the Los Angeles County Hospital by treating severe infections with vitamin C matched Dr. Klenner's enthusiasm with the remark, 'If anything should be called a miracle drug, it is vitamin C.'" [3]

The next part of this chapter will give important information on most of the known vitamins. Because of the reason discussed above, it is good to take vitamin supplements, but a vitamin supplement is no substitute for food, and neither can vitamins be assimilated without ingesting food.

The fat soluble vitamins (A,D, E, F, K)
Vitamin A
Is essential for growth of young
Increases resistance to urinary and respiratory infection
Promotes proper appetite and digestion
Is a "membrane conditioner." One of the chief functions of vitamin A is to maintain healthy skin tissues and the membranes that line all passages which open to the exterior of the body, as well as glands and their ducts.
Is necessary for proper formation and maintenance of tooth enamel and health of gums.
Assists in the proper growth of bones
Maintains proper health of sex glands and uterus
Counteracts night blindness, weak eyesight, and many eye disorders
Helps treat acne and boils when treated externally

Deficiency Symptoms:
Predisposition to colds, infections of the respiratory and urinary tract, sinusitis, abscesses in ears and mouth, general infections.
Lack of ability to see well in dim light
Acne
Rough, dry scaly skin
Sensitivity to light

Reproductive difficulties
Brittle hair

Food Sources:
Fish liver oil, fish, clams, oysters, apples, carrots, liver, green and yellow vegetables, eggs, sweet potatoes, pumpkin, squash, peppers, tomatoes, collards, kale, cheese, buttermilk, avocados, milk, yellow fruits, cantaloupe, apricots, blackberries, boysenberries, pink and red grapefruits, lemons, mangoes, nectarines, peaches, papaya, tangerines, oranges, watermelons, nuts.

Vitamin D (sunshine vitamin)
Promotes growth and proper mineralization of the bones and teeth
Essential in the formation of specific enzymes
Useful in proper gland and nerve function
Taken with A and C it can aid in preventing colds.

Deficiency Symptoms:
Poor growth and lack of normal bone development
Rickets
Osteomalacia (softening of bones in adults)
Fatigue
Arthritis
Defective teeth
Constipation
Nervousness

Food Sources:
Fish liver oils (these can be taken in capsule or liquid form), sardines, herring, salmon, tuna, milk and dairy products

Vitamin E
Absolutely essential for the adequate absorption of iron
Enhances activity of vitamin A
Protects the pituitary, adrenal and sex hormones
Prevents scar tissue formation-internally and externally
Increases the rate at which new blood vessels develop around damaged areas
Protects against muscle degeneration
Needed for blood flow to heart and lung protection
Helps regulate the pituitary gland
Retards aging
Supplies oxygen to the body
Prevents and dissolves blood clots
Alleviates fatigue
Helps alleviate leg cramps and "charley horse"

Deficiency Symptoms:
Retarded growth in children
Menstrual discomfort
Angina pectoris
Brittle and falling hair
Impotency
Miscarriage

Food Sources:
Wheat germ, soybeans, vegetable oils, broccoli, Brussels sprouts, leafy greens, spinach, whole wheat, whole-grain cereals, eggs, lettuce

Vitamin F
Aids in preventing cholesterol deposits in the arteries
Promotes healthy skin and hair
Aids in growth and well-being
Combats heart disease

Deficiency Symptoms:
Eczema
Acne

Food Sources:
Vegetables oils: wheat germ, linseed, sunflower, safflower, soybean, and peanut, sunflower seeds, peanuts, walnuts, pecans, almonds, avocados.

Vitamin K
Well known as the "coagulating factor"
Needed for blood clotting
Vital for normal liver function
Helps formation of prothrombin in the liver
Aids in reducing excessive menstrual flow
Helps to prevent internal bleeding and hemorrhages

Deficiency Symptoms:
Delayed blood clotting
Internal bleeding
Subcutaneous hemorrhage
Nose bleeds
Colitis

Food Sources:
Alfalfa, soybean oil, most green leafy vegetables, yogurt, safflower oil, fish liver oils, kelp

Water Soluble Vitamins
Vitamin C
Aids in the formation and maintenance of collagen protein. (Collagen protein is tissue "cement" for skin, cartilage, tendon and bone)
Maintains strength in blood vessels
Promotes sound healing of wounds
Influences formation of hemoglobin, absorption of iron from intestinal tract, and deposition of iron in liver tissue
Assists in the secretion of hormones from adrenals
Protects the body against infections and bacterial toxins, also against viruses
Antihistamine action
Diuretic action
Accelerates healing after surgery
Offers protection against cancer-producing agents
Lowers incidence of blood clots in veins
Aids in treatment and prevention of the common cold

Deficiency Symptoms:
Pink or hemorrhage skin follicles
Hemorrhages in the eye
Inflamed gums
Joint pains
Excessive loss of hair
In children-restlessness, irritability
Listlessness, lack of endurance
Fleeting pains in legs and joints
Small hemorrhages under skin
Gums which bleed easily

Food Sources:
All citrus fruits, berries, most green and leafy vegetables, tomatoes, cauliflower, potatoes, sweet potatoes, avocados

Vitamin B Complex(B1, B2, B3, B6, Pantothenic Acid, PABA, B12, Folic Acid, Choline, Inositol

Vitamin B-1 (Thiamine)
Known as the "morale vitamin" because of its beneficial effects on the nervous system and mental attitude
Keeps nervous system, muscles, and heart functioning normally
Assists in conversion of carbohydrates to glucose
Stabilizes the appetite
Necessary for growth, fertility, lactation

Necessary for normal function of nervous system
Aids in treatment of herpes zoster

Deficiency Symptoms:
Cardiac: palpitations, gallop rhythm, enlarged heart
Loss of ankle and knee jerk reflexes
Muscular weakness progressing to atrophy
Mental: Instability, forgetfulness, vague fears, confusion
Fatigue
Loss of appetite

Special Note:
This vitamin is present in many foods, but like all the B-vitamins, it tends to be depleted by the consumption of refined carbohydrates, alcohol, and tobacco. High temperatures also destroy this vitamin.

Food sources:
Dried yeast, whole wheat, whole ground cornmeal, whole grains. almonds, lentils, peas, tomato paste and puree, oatmeal, peanuts, most vegetables, bran, milk, potatoes, avocados, fresh orange juice, pecans, whitefish.

Vitamin B-2 (Riboflavin)
Assists the eye in light adaption
Assists in the conversion of tryptophan to niacin
Assists in the metabolism of carbohydrates, proteins and fats

Increased need in stress situations
Aids in growth and reproduction
Promotes healthy skin, nail, and hair
Helps eliminate sore mouth, lips, and tongue

Deficiency Symptoms:
Dr. Mindell says, "America's most common vitamin deficiency is riboflavin" [4]
Cracks and sores in corner of mouth
Red-purple shiny tongue
Sensation of sand on inside of eyelids
Eye fatigue, burning, itching, sensitivity to light
Capillary congestion of the sclera (white) of the eye
Cataracts
Depression

Special Note: The most common cause of B2 deficiency is poor dietary habits.

Food sources:
Leafy green vegetables, fish, eggs, milk, liver, kidney, yeast, cheese, potatoes, yogurt, avocado, pink and red salmon, almonds, peas, wild rice.

Vitamin B-3 (Niacin or Niacinamide)
It is necessary for the health of all tissue cells
Gives you healthier looking skin
Helps prevent and ease severity of migraine headaches
Helps eliminate canker sores and, often, bad breath

Helps to reduce cholesterol
Increases circulation and reduces high blood pressure
Helps nerves
It counteracts blood clotting tendencies, giving protection against coronary thrombosis, blood clots in the heart vessels (as well as against blood clots in the brain which cause stroke). Niacin is essential to growth and to the proper use of oxygen. Without it, thiamine, and riboflavin cannot function properly in the body.

Deficiency Symptoms:
Pellagra, dermatitis, diarrhea, dementia
Loss of appetite, indigestion
Small ulcers, canker sores
Schizophrenia
Burning hands and/or feet
Persons without enough niacin may develop disorders of the alimentary canal, the skin, and the nervous system.

Special Note: One of the letters to the magazine, "Let's Live" had the following letter in it, August 1980. "It is a miracle how I can be suicidal, paranoid, hallucinating–take a niacin–and it disappears!"

Food sources:
Liver, lean meat, whole-wheat products, whole-grains, brewer's yeast, kidney, wheat germ, fish,

eggs, roasted peanuts, white meat of poultry, avocados, dates, figs, prunes, potatoes, almonds, asparagus, beans, collards, mushrooms, tomato juice.

Vitamin B-6 (Pyridoxine)
Essential for the complete metabolism of many of the amino acids
Essential for the metabolism of fats
Involved in antibody production
Helps maintain sodium-potassium balance
Involved in proper DNA and RNA action
Reduces night muscle spasms, leg cramps, hand numbness
Alleviates nausea
Properly assimilates protein and fat
Helps PMS sufferers (can help regulate mood swings, irritability, fluid retention, sugar cravings and fatigue)
Helps protect against bladder cancer
Helps alleviate "carpal tunnel syndrome"

Deficiency Symptoms:
Dermatitis
Numbness of hands and feet
Green tinted urine
Dizziness, nausea, vomiting
Kidney stones
Nervous disturbances including confusion and convulsions
Anemia

Special Note: B6 is linked with hormone balance and is of special importance to women taking birth control pills. Large amounts of estrogen flooding the system when the Pill is taken can cause depression. It has been suggested that this is a result of the increased metabolism of the amino acid tryptophan which, in turn, requires more B6. Large amounts of estrogen occur naturally during pregnancy and prior to menstruation. This can lead to a bloated feeling and irritability during the menstrual cycle, or nausea and edema (water retention) during pregnancy. According to Dr. John M. Ellis, *Vitamin B6, The Doctor's Report*, all these conditions can be prevented and/or alleviated with large doses of B6 (100-200 milligrams daily).

Food sources:
Brewer's yeast, wheat bran, wheat germ, liver, kidney, heart, cantaloupe, cabbage, blackstrap molasses, milk, eggs, beef.

Vitamin B-12
Essential for normal functioning of all cells, particularly bone marrow, the nervous system, and the gastrointestinal tract
Very important in formation of nucleic acids
It is needed for red blood cell formation
Increases energy
Relieves irritability
Improves concentration, memory, and balance

Deficiency Symptoms:
Sore tongue, weakness, loss of weight
Back pains
Apathy
Pernicious anemia: anemia with degeneration of the
spinal cord

Food sources:
Liver, beef, eggs, milk, cheese, kidney, yogurt, crab,
herring, oysters, sardines, tuna, chicken, lamb, veal,
soy products, and lentil sprouts.

Vitamin B5 Pantothenic Acid
Helps in cell building, maintaining normal growth,
and development of the central nervous system
Aids in wound healing
Fights infection by building antibodies
Prevents fatigue

Deficiency Symptoms:
Fatigue, headache, personality changes
Dizziness, rapid heart rate on exertion
Gastric distress, constipation
Numbness or tingling of hands and feet
Burning sensation of hands and feet
Tendency toward hypoglycemia, arthritis

Food sources:
Whole grains, wheat germ, bran, meat, liver, heart, green vegetables, brewer's yeast, nuts, chicken, crude molasses, yogurt, tuna, apricots, avocados, dates, watermelon, barley, rice, broccoli, cauliflower, kale, mushrooms, green peas, sweet potatoes.

Biotin
Essential in the formation of nucleic acids
Essential in the formation of glycogen
Helps in preventive treatment for baldness
Aids in keeping hair from turning gray
Eases muscle pains
Alleviates eczema and dermatitis
Keep in mind that biotin works synergistically and more effectively with B2, B6, niacin and A

Deficiency Symptoms:
Dermatitis and sore tongue
Loss of appetite and nausea
Low-grade anemia
Insomnia
Muscle pain
Intense depression
Extreme exhaustion

Food Sources:
Nuts, fruits, brewer's yeast, beef liver, egg yolk, milk, kidney, unpolished rice, mushrooms, corn, legumes, and cauliflower.

Choline
Aids in metabolism of fats
It assists normal nerve function
Assists in the synthesis of certain hormones
Works with inositol to utilize fats and cholesterol
One of the few substances able to penetrate the blood-brain barrier, which goes directly into the brain cells to produce a chemical that aids memory
Assists in conquering memory loss
Is often referred to as "brain food"

Deficiency Symptoms:
Fatty degeneration of liver
Heart muscle lesions
Hemmorrhagic lesions in kidneys
Arteriosclerosis

Food Sources:
Fish, egg yolks, soybeans, brain, heart, green leafy vegetables, yeast, liver, wheat germ, lecithin, eggplant.

Inositol
Aids in metabolism of fats
Helps lower cholesterol levels
Promotes healthy hair and aids in preventing fallout
Helps prevent eczema

Deficiency Symptoms:
Atherosclerosis
Excema

Food sources:
Liver, brewer's yeast, dried lima beans, beef brains and heart, cantaloupe, grapefruit, raisins, wheat germ, unrefined molasses, peanuts, cabbage.

Folic Acid
Necessary for synthesis of nucleic acids
Necessary for synthesis of certain amino acids
Prevention of macrocytic anemia
Utilization of amino acids
Essential to the formation of red blood cells
Protects against intestinal parasites and food poisoning
May delay hair graying when used in conjunction with pantothenic acid and PABA
Acts as a preventive for canker sores
Helps ward off anemia

Deficiency Symptoms:
Macrocytic anemia: lack of mature red blood cells
Smooth, red tongue
Gastrointestinal disturbances, diarrhea

Food sources:
Brewers Yeast, Wheat Germ, Soy flour, Garbanzo beans, Deep green leafy vegetables, carrots, egg yolk,

cantaloupe, apricots, pumpkin, avocados, beans, whole wheat and dark rye flour, Wheat Bran, potatoes.

Para-Aminobenzoic (PABA)
Helps to prevent excema and loss of pigmentation
High amounts are effective in burn pain control
Facilitates the body's production of folic acid
Acts as a part of the coenzyme system
Keeps skin healthy and smooth
Helps to restore natural color to hair

Deficiency Symptoms:
Gastrointestinal disorders
Fatigue, irritability, depression
Pigmentation loss in skin in patches
Lupus Erythematosus
Eczema

Food Sources:
Liver, brewer's yeast, kidney, whole grains, rice, bran, wheat germ, molasses, avocados, bananas, blackberries, cantaloupe, dates, nectarines, strawberries, oatmeal, shredded wheat, almonds, pecans, peas, beans.

B-15 (Pangamic Acid)
Keeps fat from infiltrating the liver
Serves as a detoxification agent
Increases the body's efficiency in using oxygen

Regulates blood levels of steroids
Extends cell lifespan
Lower blood cholesterol level

Deficiency Symptoms:
Premature aging
Asthma, emphysema
Cirrhosis, hepatitis, jaundice of the liver
Fatigue
Heart palpitation, angina pains

Food Sources:
Brewer's yeast, whole brown rice, whole grains, pumpkin seeds, sesame seeds.

*You will notice that yeast was mentioned as being one of the food sources of many of the above vitamins. Look in chapter 16 to understand what kinds of yeast these are.

Remember, all foods listed above, except animal products, should be eaten while they are fresh and in their raw, natural state, as much as possible. Nuts should be unsalted and without oil, vegetables should be steamed or eaten raw so that vitamin content will be at their maximum strength.

Everyday, except when fasting, I take my handful of vitamins after my morning meal. If you take 1 Beta Carotene (vitamin A) 25,000 IU, 1 Total B vitamin, which contains the whole B family properly balanced, 1 Vitamin E (in either dry or fat form) 400-800 IU, 1 Garlic capsule, 1 Lecithin capsule, 1 Multiple Mineral capsule, 4-6 Spirulina tablets, among other things, which you will discover when you start studying about the wonderful world of nutrition and its connection with the body, you will definitely start feeling better.

I also take my vitamin C in granulated form. Each morning before breakfast I mix 2 Tablespoons of brewer's yeast, 1 Tablespoon of apple cider vinegar (purchased at the health store), and 1/2-1 teaspoon of ascorbic acid in 1/2 cup of apple or grape juice and drink it. It does not taste that good, but the benefits are incredible (see chapter 16).

Chapter 4

The
Mighty Minerals

*V*itamins are important, but they can do nothing for the body without minerals. Dr. Mindell says he likes to call minerals the Cinderella's of the nutrition world, because, "though very few people are aware of it, vitamins cannot function, cannot be assimilated, without the aid of minerals. And though the body can synthesize some vitamins, it cannot manufacture a *single* mineral." [1]

Some mineral supplements are available in chelated form, which means that the minerals are attached to a protein molecule that transports them to the bloodstream in order to enhance their absorption. When mineral supplements are taken with a meal, they are usually automatically chelated in the stomach during digestion.

Calcium
Balances potassium and sodium for muscle tone
Necessary for heartbeat regulation
Assists in blood clotting
Required for normal nerve transmission
Maintains strong bones and healthy teeth
Alleviates insomnia
Helps metabolize your body's iron
Aids the nervous system

Deficiency Symptoms:
Poor quality of bones and teeth
Osteoporosis
Leg Cramps
Excessive and lengthy menstruation
Nervousness, irritability

Food Sources:
Milk and milk products, all cheeses, soybeans, sardines, salmon, peanuts, walnuts, sunflower seeds, beans, green vegetables (mustard greens, broccoli, and kale), yogurt, shellfish, egg yolk, tofu, turnips, dates, almonds, blackstrap molasses, kale, peas, mustard greens.

Phosphorus
Phosphorus has been called the brain power of the mineral world. It makes lecithin. (White sugar destroys phosphorus)
Formation of strong bones and teeth
Involved in virtually all physiological chemical reactions
Important for heart regularity
Essential for normal kidney functioning
Provides energy and vigor

Deficiency Symptoms:
Mental and physical fatigue
Irregular breathing
Poor bone and tooth structure
Arthritis
Rickets, pyorrhea

Food Sources:
Fish, poultry, meat, whole grains, eggs, nuts, yogurt, cereals, legumes and seeds

Potassium
Acts as a stimulant to the kidneys
Assists in conversion of glucose to glycogen
Necessary for normal health of adrenals
Aids in clear thinking by sending oxygen to the brain
Helps dispose of body wastes
Assists in reducing blood pressure
Aids in allergy treatment

Is essential for healthy glands
Is essential to fight against hypoglycemia
Adequate potassium is necessary for normal sugar metabolism (Diabetic persons are often deficient in potassium)

Deficiency Symptoms:
Muscular Weakness
Edema
Nervousness
Hypoglycemia
Insufficient potassium causes cardiac abnormalities and a slow, weak, irregular pulse

Food Sources:
Citrus fruits, cantaloupe, tomatoes, watercress, all green leafy vegetables, sunflower seeds, bananas, potatoes, fish, poultry, cereals, whole-grains, almonds, raisins, peanuts, dates, avocados, pecans, halibut, spinach, mushrooms, broccoli, and legumes

Sodium
Regulates the internal fluid pH
With potassium, regulates the body fluids
Aids in preventing sunstroke
Helps nerves and muscles to function properly

Deficiency Symptoms:
Dehydration

Food Sources:
Sea Salt, shellfish, carrots, beets, artichokes, dried beef, brains, kidney

Chlorine
Regulates the blood's alkaline acid balance
Aids in digestion
Helps keep you limber
Helps liver to function

Deficiency Symptoms:
Loss of hair and teeth

Food Sources:
Sea Salt, kelp, olives

Magnesium
Essential for maintenance of DNA and RNA
Necessary for normal contraction of muscles
Essential for effective nerve and muscle functioning
Known as the "antistress mineral"
Aids in fighting depression
Promotes a healthier cardiovascular system and helps prevent heart attacks
Keeps teeth healthier
Helps prevent calcium deposits, kidney stones, and gallstones
Brings relief from indigestion

Deficiency Symptoms:
Excessive irritability of nerves and muscles
Nervous tics and twitches (B6 also involved)
Irregular heart beat
Convulsions and seizures

Food Sources:
Figs, lemons, grapefruit, yellow corn, almonds, nuts, seeds, dark green vegetables, apples, potatoes, soy, whole grains, and seaweed

    *In *Let's Live* magazine, November 1995 issue, Dr. Earl Mindell, R.Ph., Ph, D., says that a chronic magnesium deficiency is likely partially responsible for America's high rate of heart disease, and a recent study indicates it may be closely linked to migraine headaches.

    He recommends everyone take at least 300 mg of magnesium daily, and older Americans should take 600 mg to 800 mg daily to help with calcium absorption.

Iron
Necessary for the production of hemoglobin (red blood corpuscles)
Copper, cobalt, manganese, and vitamin C are necessary to assimilate iron
Aids growth
Promotes resistance to disease
Prevents fatigue

Cure and prevent iron-deficiency anemia
Bring back good skin tone

Deficiency Symptoms:
Anemia, pale skin, abnormal fatigue
Shortness of breath
Lack of appetite

Food Sources:
Liver, beef kidney, heart, farina, raw clams, dried apricots, prunes and peaches, egg yolks, oysters, nuts, beans, asparagus, molasses, oatmeal, potatoes, seaweed, cherries, tuna, raisins, peanuts, whole wheat bread

Manganese
Proper utilization of glucose
Normal pancreas function and development
Prevention of sterility
Helps eliminate fatigue
Aids in Muscle reflexes
Improves memory
Reduces nervous irritability

Deficiency Symptoms:
Weakness of ligaments and tendons

Food Sources:
Nuts, green leafy vegetables, peas, beets, egg yolks, whole grain cereals, carrots, celery, pineapple, liver

Iodine
Helps regulate any metabolic functions in the body
Helpful in thyroid (Two-thirds of the body's iodine is in the thyroid gland)
Helps by burning excess fat
Promotes proper growth
Gives energy
Improves mental alacrity
Promotes healthy hair, nails, skin, and teeth

Deficiency Symptoms:
Goiter
Slow mental reactions
Dry hair, brittle nails
Obesity

Food Sources:
Kelp, vegetables grown in iodine-rich soil, onions, all seafood, mushrooms

Fluorine
Increases deposition of calcium
Reduces tooth decay
Strengthens bones

Deficiency Symptoms:
Poor tooth development

Food Sources:
Seafood, gelatin

Copper
Facilitates iron absorption
Involved in protein metabolism and the healing process
Assists the body to oxidize vitamin C
Necessary for production of RNA
Keeps your energy up by aiding in effective iron absorption

Deficiency Symptoms:
General weakness, anemia
Impaired respiration
Skin sores

Food Sources:
Dried beans, peas, whole wheat, prunes, calf and beef liver, shrimp, most seafood

Cobalt
Is an integral part of vitamin B12
Essential for red blood cells
Helps prevent anemia

Deficiency Symptom:
Anemia

Food Sources:
Meat, kidney, liver, milk, oysters, clams

Chromium
Stimulates enzymes involved in glucose metabolism
Increases effectiveness of insulin
Helps bring protein where it is needed
Aids growth
Helps prevent and lower high blood pressure
Works as a deterrent for diabetes

Deficiency Symptoms:
A suspected factor in arteriosclerosis and diabetes

Food Sources:
Meat, shellfish, chicken, corn oil, clams, brewer's yeast

Zinc
Necessary for absorption and activity of vitamins, particularly B-complex
Helps in the formation of insulin
Helpful in healing wounds and burns
Necessary for normal prostate function
Gets rid of white spots on fingernails
Aids in treatment of infertility
Helps avoid prostate problems
Promotes growth and mental alertness

Deficiency Symptoms:
Increased fatigue
Susceptibility to infection
Loss of taste and smell sensitivity

Food Sources:
Round steak, lamb chops, wheat germ, brewer's yeast, pumpkin seeds, eggs, nonfat dry milk, ground mustard

Selenium
Aids in keeping youthful elasticity in tissues
Alleviates hot flashes and menopausal distress
Helps in treatment and prevention of dandruff
Possibly neutralizes certain carcinogens and provides protection from some cancers

Deficiency Symptoms:
Premature stamina loss

Food Sources:
Wheat germ, bran, tuna fish, onions, tomatoes, broccoli, organ meats, seafood, whole grains, brown rice, garlic, cabbage, chicken, eggs

Sulfur
Essential for healthy hair, skin, and nails
Tones up skin and makes hair more lustrous
Helps fight bacterial infections

Helps maintain oxygen balance necessary for proper brain function
Aids the liver in bile secretion

Deficiency Symptoms:
Brittle Nails
Splitting Hair
Difficulty focusing the eyes
Itchy skin, especially around the nose and mouth

Food Sources:
Lean Beef, dried beans, fish, eggs, cabbage, eggs, broccoli, Brussels sprouts, cauliflower

Vanadium
Inhibits the formation of cholesterol in blood vessels
Aids in preventing heart attacks

Deficiency Symptoms:
None known

Food Source:
Fish

Molybdenum
Assists in mobilizing iron
Helps in preventing anemia
Promotes general well-being

Deficiency Symptoms:
None known

Food Sources:
Dark green leafy vegetables, whole grains, legumes (beans and peas, etc.).

Silicon
Needed for normal growth and bone development
Beauty mineral

Food Sources:
Steel-cut oats, Apples, honey, avocados, artichokes, sunflower seeds, alfalfa, high-fiber foods, vegetables, grains.

Many foods can sometimes be depleted in rich minerals due to soil depletion; therefore, the body is fed inferior foods lacking the proper minerals. Dr. Charles Northen said, "I'm an M.D., my work lies in the field of biochemistry and nutrition. I gave up medicine because there is a wider and more important work. Sick soils mean sick plants, sick animals, and sick people. Physical, mental, and moral fitness depends largely upon an ample supply and a proper proportion of the minerals in our food." [2]

There are at least 16 minerals the body needs to maintain good health. They are found in the muscles, brain, glands, heart, hair, and blood. The body is constantly excreting them and they can only be restored by the diet or food supplements, and need to be constantly replenished.

Most of the minerals are found in sea products. That is why seaweed nutrients such as kelp, nori, and dulse are so valuable. The late Paul Bragg, an amazing healthy older man who stayed incredibly physically fit said he made seaweed products a part of his diet everyday. One reason seaweeds are so helpful is that they include not only minerals, but vitamins and protein factors as well. Dr. Melchior T. Dikkers, Ph.D., a director of a trace mineral research laboratory says, "Some seaweeds contain more vitamin A and D than cod liver oil. They contain all the B-complex vitamins, vitamin C, and vitamin E. In fact all of the vitamins and minerals are found in larger amounts in seaweed than in any land vegetation. The proportion of minerals is almost identical with that in the human blood."

Dr. Dikkers lists the following assets of seaweed:

- It has antibiotic qualities.
- It helps to relieve constipation and soothes intestinal irritation.
- It has been used for hundreds of years for diarrhea and dysentery.
- Seaweed extracts were used for the relief of respiratory irritations due to poisonous gas during World War I.
- It promotes marked improvement in arthritic cases.

- It provides relief of eye conditions, such as iritis and cataract.
- It increases sense of well being.

Murray Rose, the great swimmer, and the youngest three-time gold medal winner of the Olympics, made Irish moss, rich in protein, minerals, and some vitamins, one of the mainstays of his diet during his training. He felt it was an important part in maintaining his stamina during the Olympics, as he explained in the book *Faith, Love and Seaweed.*

If you are not one that enjoys eating the paper thin seaweed which is used to wrap Japanese special food preparations, or sprinkle it in your soup, etc., then you can do as I do, take kelp in tablet form.

Chapter 5

Protein, Fats, Carbohydrates, and Cholesterol

Linda A. Clark, M.A. states in her book, *Secrets of Health and Beauty,* that "Protein is the essential stuff of which all living tissue is made. Protein cannot be stored in the body very long. When the supply is depleted the body is forced to feed on itself. Prolonged shortage of protein can cause anemia, kidney disease, liver disease, peptic ulcer, poor wound healing, lack of resistance to infection, irritability, fatigue, low blood pressure, weakness, poor circulation, constipation, edema (water storage) or poor vision." [1]

The word protein coined by a Dutch chemist in 1839 means "*of first importance*". It is the stuff of life: no protein, no life. The need for protein in the function of the following body parts exemplifies the importance of protein.

- To function properly the liver needs protein; it must also receive all the amino acids at one time.
- The hormone, a chemical regulator, is a protein.
- The genes, the controller of heredity, are protein.
- The secretion of the thyroid gland is a protein.
- Insulin, produced by the pancreas, is a protein.
- The secretions of the pituitary gland, the master gland of the body, are proteins.
- Antibodies, which defend the body against infection, are proteins.
- All enzymes, which control a multitude of body functions, are proteins.
- Hemoglobin, the red coloring matter of the blood, is protein.
- If you have a wound, a cut, or a burn, protein is lost in the fluid which escapes. The remaking of healthy tissue over an injury of the body must have protein to repair the damage.
- Your muscles, including your liver, kidneys, and especially your heart, to even your eyes, are made of protein.
- Lack of protein weakens muscles tone and makes them flabby. Without it your facial muscles will began to drop and your skin will shrivel and wither. Wrinkles and premature aging will appear.
- Your hair is 97% protein, and 3% ash.

What kind of protein is best (animal vs. vegetable)? More recent information suggests vegetable protein-diet has great potential to reduce cholesterol, heart disease and pain, while animal protein is being re-evaluated as to its benefits, and its contribution to the development of disease and pain. Also people may not need as much protein as thought (especially as one grows older).

Dr. Michael Murray, leading researcher in the field of natural medicine, in his interview on *Healthline*, May 16, 1995, related facts concerning the China diet study. In China, they took 6,500 Chinese for six years and compared average Americans' diet to that of the rural Chinese. In the findings they found that in America many were taking nearly 100 grams of protein a day and the Chinese were taking 60 grams a day, but only 4 percent came from animal products, while the Americans were taking in 70% from animal products, animal fat, and animal protein. The results spoke for themselves. In China, osteroporous was virtually unknown, female cancers were way down, while earlier menstrual cycles for Americans were way up, which means more breast and cervical cancer.

Most nutritionists agree that 55-65 grams of protein are the recommended amount. Some plant proteins are preferable to others. Linda Clark, M.A. states, "The U.S. Department of Agriculture rates the protein content of sunflower seeds almost as high as steak, and higher than all other vegetable seeds. Its protein is 98 per cent digestible, with a utilization value of 64.5 per cent, which places the seeds in the same classification as egg protein...The best sources of vegetable proteins are legumes (certain peas and beans), seeds, some grasses, and some nuts. The soybean is the most complete protein of all vegetables." [2]

Protein is what makes you. There are 3 billion cells in your body that are being rebuilt every minute. Protein shapes your body, builds up your hair, beautifies your skin. Protein deficiency can even cause your hair to turn gray. Your hair is 97% protein, the rest is ash.

Protein Foods:	Amount	Grams of Protein
Some of these foods are better for you than others.		
Wheat Germ	1/2 cup	24grams
Brewer's Yeast	1/2 cup	50grams
Beef	Average helping	17
Chicken	Average helping	18
Heart	Average helping	11
Kidney	Average helping	11
Lamb chop	1 medium	10
Liver	Average helping	19
Turkey	Average helping	21
Milk, dried skim	1/2 cup	53
Yogurt	1qt.	33
Cheese	1 piece	12
2x1x1inches		

Cottage cheese	3 tbs.	10
Cream cheese	11/2 tbs.	8
Egg	1	6
Salmon, canned	1/3 cup	22
Tuna fish, canned	2 Tbs.	12
Peanuts	2 tbs.	10
Peanut flour	1 cup	59
Peanut butter	2 tbs.	14
Walnuts	1/2 cup	8
Pecans	10 meats	3
Lima beans	1/2 cup	8
Navy beans	1/2 cup	6
Soybeans,dried	1/2 cup	51
Soya flour	1 cup	37
Lentils	1/2 cup	9
Peas, dried	1/2	7
Barley, whole	1/2 cup cooked	8
Buckwheat, whole	1/3 cup	12
Rice, brown	3/4 cup	3
Shredded wheat	1 biscuit	3
Wheat germ	1/2 cup	24
Yeast, dried	1 tbs.	4

Some people feel that meat consumption is needed for proteins. Do other foods contain proteins? Since proteins are such vital and important nutrients, it is helpful to know that God in His infinite wisdom has made protein a part of almost every natural food available to man. Every plant, every vegetable, every seed or nut contains some protein. It is practically impossible to eat a natural food without eating some protein.

The protein quality in some of the vegetables sources is even superior to the meat protein, as in the case of protein from soybeans, some nuts (cashews, almonds), potatoes and green vegetables. Plain baked potatoes are a good source of complete proteins. Such foods as soybeans, sesame seeds, many nuts, millet, potatoes, and green vegetables all contain complete proteins, as good or better than meat proteins, without meat's undesirable side effects.

Spirulina is one of nature's original whole foods and is higher in protein than any other natural food. Spirulina is a complete protein, providing all 21 amino acids, including the essential amino acids. It contains approximately 13 grams of protein in two tablespoons full. Far more nutritious than any known food, Spirulina also contains the entire B-complex. It is rich in carotene (vitamin A precursor), and in minerals and fatty acids. Spirulina contains almost twice as much B12 per gram as dried liver which was considered the richest source of this nutrient. Spirulina is rich in the minerals iron, phosphorus, zinc, potassium, magnesium, and contains twenty-six times the calcium of milk. It also contains the trace minerals selenium and chromium.

The following amounts are suggested in a "Consumer Information" bulletin released by one Spirulina distributor.

If consuming regular meals:		
3 grams (by weight) per day		
If consuming just liquids:		
30 grams (by weight) per day		
1 tablet	=	1/2 gram
1 tsp. powder	=	3 grams
1T. powder	=	10 grams

Protein is a chemical compound that is an essential part of every cell. All living things must have proteins to stay alive. Proteins repair damaged cells, build new tissues, and do many other vital jobs. All proteins contain the chemicals carbon, hydrogen, nitrogen, and oxygen. Some proteins also contain sulfur or phosphorus.

Structure of Proteins: Proteins consist of many units called amino acids linked together in long chains. Amino acids are organic acids that contain nitrogen. The individual chains, called peptides, either lie straight, or coiled like a spring. At intervals along their lengths, they are linked to other peptide chains to form the complex network of peptides that makes up a protein.

Proteins are digested in the stomach and small intestine, and are absorbed into the blood as amino acids. The amino acids are carried to all organs and tissues, where they are used to build new cells.

A single protein molecule may contain many hundreds of each of about 20 kinds of amino acids. The total number of amino acids, and the order in which the acids are arranged vary from protein to protein.

Proteins furnish "building blocks" for the body. The body does not store protein. That is why it is important to eat some protein foods every day. Too little protein in your diet makes the muscles soft and flabby. The body also uses protein for energy if a person does not eat enough carbohydrates and fats.

Proteins are important for growth, development, and maintenance of life. They are *protective foods*. They satisfy hunger, stick to the ribs, nourish, and keep the body young and elastic.

In addition to building and repairing body tissue, protein is used in making hemoglobin, the iron-containing substance of the red blood corpuscles. Hormones are made of proteins. All of the enzymes in the body, which aid in the production of energy, the digestion of foods, the building of new tissue, and the tearing down of worn-out tissue, are made of protein. Proteins in the blood are responsible for the collection of urine and waste from the tissues. Proteins also help prevent the blood and tissues from becoming either too acid or too alkaline. They are important in making possible the clotting of the blood. Proteins even form substances known as antibodies, which combine with and render harmless the bacteria, bacterial toxins, and other foreign materials. Protein is an "active" nutrient, busily employed in repairing the daily wear and tear.

According to Linda A. Clark, M.A., in her book *Secrets of Health and Beauty,* prolonged protein deficiency, however, can cause the following disturbances:

Anemia
Kidney disease
Liver disease
Peptic ulcer
Poor wound healing
Lack of resistance to infection
Irritability
Fatigue
Low blood pressure
Weakness
High cholesterol
Poor circulation
Constipation
Mental retardation in children
Edema (water storage)
Poor vision

Fats

Gayelord Hauser, health counselor, describes the body like this: "As a simplified, perhaps crude, illustration, think of your body as a motor car. It is made of protein, inside and out. Arteries, glands, colon, connective tissue; muscles, skin, bones, hair, teeth, eyes: all contain protein and are maintained and rebuilt with protein. Fats and carbohydrates are your body's oil and gasoline; they are burned together to produce energy. Vitamins and minerals are its spark plugs, essential to the utilization of food and its assimilation into the blood stream." [3]

"Fat is used as a source of sustained energy, as heat insulation under the skin, as a padding for the framework, and to round out the contours of the body. Fat foods supply more than twice the number of calories available from the same amount of protein or carbohydrate...Fat is more slowly digested and absorbed than all other foodstuffs...When liquid vegetable fats are used in normal amounts, they are completely and easily digested. Unfortunately, with increased prosperity, Americans, instead of using 25 percent fat in their daily meals, today consume 40 to 50 percent of their calories in hard fats...Hard animal fats do create a high cholesterol level in the blood. The liquid golden vegetable oils do not." [4]

Author's note: The preceding paragraph was first written in 1951 and revised in 1974. Since then, there has been much written on the *good* fats and the *bad* fats.

Liquid vegetable oils contain the unsaturated fatty acids (especially linoleic acid, which is so important not only for good health, but for good looks). "A German chemist, in his experiments with animals, proved that when he deprived his animals of linoleic acid, their skin became dry and scaly and their hair became dry and thin. As soon as the important linoleic acid was returned to the diet, the skin and hair again became normal." [5]

Noted nutrition expert, Linda Clark, recommends taking two tablespoons of the liquid vegetable oils such as safflower, olive, sunflower, etc. To maintain good health one should avoid hydrogenated fats such as hydrogenated peanut butter, processed cheeses, solid cooking fats and French-fried foods cooked in these solid fats. Use unrefined, or cold-pressed oils for best results. A good way to include the oils in your daily diet is to use them in salad dressings.

Health counselor, Siri Khalsa, writes in the 1995, Vol. XIX, No. 12 "Nutrition News," the following: "Fats and fatlike substances are called *lipids*. They are essential to health. The three major types of interest to us are triglycerides, phospholipids, and cholesterol...Found in every cell, they are integrally involved in cell membrane structure, blood and tissue structure, enzyme reactions, the synthesis and use of sterol hormones, and the hormone-like prostaglandins, plus they are imperative to memory and nervous system functions.

"*Triglycerides* are what we commonly refer to as fat. They comprise 95 percent of the lipids in foods. When we eat them, they are digested and then reformed into triglycerides again. These circulate in the blood as they as they are taken up for various functions. Their principal use is as an energy source for metabolism, a function shared almost equally with carbohydrates.

"*Phospholipids* are the second class of lipids, and many kinds exist in the body, especially in the brain. Lecithin is a phosopholipid. It is found in the cells; it is part of the fat digestion process; and it is an emulsifying phospholipid. The presence of lecithin makes it possible for fats and water to mix.

"Although *cholesterol*, has a very different structure from the triglycerides and phospholipds, it is likewise not water soluble. Cholesterol is essential to life. It is too much cholesterol which presents a health problem. It is a constituent of cell membranes and nerve fibers, bile, the sex hormones, and vitamin D. Found in all body tissues, it is particularly concentrated in the liver, blood, and the brain."

In January, 1989, Artesian Health Store of Stockton, California, issued a list of eighteen items which lower cholesterol. They are the following:

1.   *Apples* eaten on a daily basis have been shown in various studies here and in Europe to lower blood serum cholesterol by approximately 10 percent. Various researchers put test subjects on two to three apples a day. In an apple eating experiment by French researcher, R. Sable-Amplis, of the University of Paul Sabatier-eighty percent of the group eating two to three apples daily showed reduced cholesterol within a month, about a 10 percent decline. HDL, the good guy cholesterol rose, and the bad guy LDL cholesterol dropped.

2.   *"Barley* is a star at reducing blood serum cholesterol levels," says Dr. Asaf Qureshi, a scientist in the U.S. Dept. of Agriculture's Cereal Crops Research Unit in Madison, Wisconsin. Dr. Qureshi feels that barley scores by lowering the liver's ability to produce cholesterol. It can be used several times a week as a cooked cereal or in baked good: breads or muffins.

3.   *Beans* (pinto or navy). As little each day as one cooked cup lowered cholesterol by 19 percent in subjects tested by Dr. James Anderson, fiber expert at the University of Kentucky. Also the ratio of HDL to LDL became more favorable. (Even baked beans help. No sugar, please! Use honey, maple syrup, or molasses.)

4.   *Carrots* (three medium size raw, eaten daily) have been shown to lower cholesterol by almost eleven percent.

5.   *Cauliflower,* which is rich in fiber, promotes bowel regularity and decreases blood cholesterol, while also discouraging cancer.

6.   *Eggplant*: At the University of Texas, researchers found that eggplant serves a special function in cholesterol control. Eggplant appears to block blood levels of cholesterol from rising when fatty foods have been eaten.

7.   *Figs* (dried) have been shown to flush out excess cholesterol.

8.   *Lecithin* (derived from soybeans): slightly more than one ounce daily reduced blood levels of cholesterol by 18 percent.

9.   *Oat Bran*, a water soluble fiber, is one of the most effective foods for reducing cholesterol. A study reported in the *Journal of the American Medical Association* revealed that eating oat bran daily as a cereal or in muffins can reduce blood cholesterol by up to 19 percent.

10.   *Olive Oil*, as demonstrated by Dr. Scott M. Grundy, of the Center for Human Nutrition at the University of Texas in Dallas, can lower or control cholesterol levels.   Grundy takes two teaspoonfuls daily and reduces his consumption of fats.

11.   *Prunes* contain various types of fiber and as few as three large ones daily can lower cholesterol appreciably.

12.   *Fish and Fish Oils*, known for their EPA and DHA (Omega 3) content, have received much attention lately for their value in helping to reduce fat and cholesterol levels in the blood.   A number of good studies indicate that eating fish several times a week and/or supplementation with Omega-3 capsules will cause the body to produce more of the beneficial high-density lipoproteins (HDL) which help to lower cholesterol and triglyceride levels.

13.   *Soybeans* and products derived from them (soy milk, lecithin, and tofu), help break down fatty deposits so they can be flushed from the body

more readily and, in the process, also lowers blood cholesterol. Soybean products seem to work best on patients with extra high cholesterol, 300 or more. Researchers at the University of Milan, Italy, caused cholesterol levels to plummet by fifteen to twenty percent, simply by having patients eat soybean products in place of meat and milk products.

14. *Garlic* has been shown to lower blood serum cholesterol by nearly 10% in 25 days. An Indian researcher, Dr. M. Sucur, fed several cloves per day to 200 volunteers. Cholesterol dropped in almost all of this group with high serum levels. (Garlic capsules can accomplish the same thing).

15. *Sweet Potatoes* contain water soluble fiber and beta-carotene. Both contribute in lowering cholesterol. In a Japanese study, sweet potato fiber proved the best of 28 fruit and vegetable fibers for binding cholesterol and removing it.

16. *Vitamin C.* It was shown in a recent study conducted in Scotland that just 1000 mg of Vitamin C daily helped to reduce cholesterol levels (*Scotland Medical Journal*, 1989).

17. *Niacin.* Still another substance making news for its ability to help lower cholesterol, especially LDL cholesterol, is the Vitamin B, niacin.

18. *Exercise.* Researcher Josef Patsch, at Baylor College of Medicine, found that daily exercise is one of the best means of lowering blood serum cholesterol. This is no quick fix. The program must be continued regularly, insists Patsch.

Carbohydrates

The chief function of carbohydrates is to provide energy for the body, for brain function, and for muscular exertion. They also assist in the digestion and assimilation of other foods. Carbohydrates are essential to health, but over consumption of them is stored as fat. Another minus factor of excessive carbohydrate intake is that it causes B vitamin deficiency.

The best carbohydrates are found chiefly in whole grains, nuts, seeds, vegetables and fruits, such as potatoes, bananas, etc.. Nutritionists suggest that at least 1 gram of carbohydrate daily for each 3 pounds of ideal body weight is the minimum necessary for proper body function.

Gayelord Hauser, health counselor, writes the following: "You never need to worry about not getting enough sugar...Practically every mouthful of fruit and vegetables you eat contains sugar. All breads, cereals, dried beans, and other starchy vegetables are changed to sugar in the process of digestion." [6]

The best sweeteners are unheated honey, unsulphured molasses, maple sugar, natural brown sugar, and unsulphured dried fruit. There is nothing much more delicious than a slice of homemade bread, buttered and dripping with clover honey. Dr. John Yudkin made the statement to the Select Committee on Nutrition and Human Needs, during the sessions aired between April 30-May 2, 1973. He said that sugar is the only available food that provides calories free from any trace of nutrients. He explained that the human being can make all the glucose (blood sugar) it needs from rather small amounts of other dietary carbohydrates, mostly starches, and from parts of the protein and fat that we eat.

Honey vs. Sugar:

Nature intended that we have a trickle of sugar passing through the intestinal walls at all times, and one teaspoon of sugar in our bloodstream of all times. In honey, the sugar has already been digested in the bee's stomach. Honey therefore combines two natural sugars, dextrose and levelose, which enter the blood stream immediately. Free from bacteria, and non-irritating to the digestive track, honey is, of all sugars, handled best by the kidneys. It is rich is many vital minerals taken from the flowers and plants. By an infallible instinct, the bee chooses only those flowers which are highest in quality, manufacturing a perfect food derived only from the healthiest plants. Honey provides a quick energy release and is packed with nutrients the body needs to build and rebuild itself.

Ordinary white sugar and honey differ nutritionally in every way. According to the U.S. Department of Agriculture's food composition tables, a pound of granulated white sugar, either cane or beet, contains nothing but carbohydrates and calories. Everything else is removed in processing: all protein, minerals, and vitamins present in the raw material.

One pound is left containing 451.7 total carbohydrates and 1,748 calories. Extracted or strained honey contains some of every major nutrient except vitamin A. Included in one pound of honey are: 1.4 grams of proteins, 3 milligrams of calcium, 73 milligrams of phosphorous, 4.1 milligrams of iron, .02 milligrams of riboflavin, 1.0 milligrams of niacin, 16 milligrams of vitamin C 260.9 total carbohydrate, and 1,333 calories.

Special Note: Wise Solomon penned these words. "My son, eat thou honey, because it is good; and the honeycomb, which is sweet to thy taste" (Proverbs 24:13), but it should be in small amounts. "It is not good to eat much honey" (Proverbs 25:27).

Chapter 6

Healthy Skin and Hair

The skin is the body's protection against dirt and foreign substances of every kind. It heals and renews itself, day in and day out. The skin needs nourishishment and that comes from within. There is no part of the body that can thrive without good nutrition, and the skin needs good life-giving elements. First, the skin needs the proteins, the building blocks out of which new cells are made. Secondly, the skin needs the full list of minerals, especially iron, which gives the blood its power to carry a full load of oxygen. Your skin needs a constant supply of oxygen so that the red blood flowing through the capillaries close to the surface, can give your skin its live, glowing radiance.

The third thing the skin needs are vitamins: Vitamin A, to preserve smooth texture and avoid drying and roughness, all the B vitamins to keep the skin youthful and firm, to prevent excessive oiliness, to keep the color clear and free from pigmentation (the B vitamins are the best, most direct route to a luminous complexion); and vitamin C, for elasticity and also for resistance to infection. Vitamin C is a number one beauty secret. It helps to keep collagen elastic and strong. Vitamin C deficient collagen is mostly responsible for the early appearance of wrinkles.

What goes inside the body is going to show up on the outside in the quality of your skin. Some foods are enhancing, while some are destroying.

Gayelord Hauser tells how the Chinese people in general have handsome, thick, black hair as long as they stick to their native diet. "They rarely suffer from baldness, and their hair keeps its blue-black color until late in life. Inheritance? No doubt, but it is also true that the Chinese cuisine is very high in minerals and many B vitamins. They eat quantities of soybeans and soy sauce and a great variety of vegetables, and their diet is so rich in first class proteins such as fish and sea food. They also consume quantities of iodine-rich sea greens of all kinds. The Chinese never overcook their vegetables, they never throw away the cooking water, and their cooking fat is liquid vegetable oil, rich with the unsaturated fatty acids. You never find hardened fat in a Chinese household.

"The Chinese and Sicilian diets are both rich in B vitamins. I am convinced that the vitamins of the B complex are important for the health, beauty, and even the color of the hair. Scientists have been able to prove in animal experiments that there are three so-called anti-gray factors. They are called pantothenic acid, para-aminobenzoic acid, and choline." [7]

Glayelord Hauser shares in his book, *Look Younger-Live Longer,* some interesting information about the thyroid gland and its effect on beauty. This gland lies in the foreground of the throat, astride the windpipe, and has been called the "watchman" between the physical and mental body. Mr. Hauser says the thyroid secretes a liquid which is constantly poured into the blood stream and carried to all parts of the body, and removal or disability of the thyroid can turn a youthful person into an old one.

One of the important functions of the thyroid is the burning of fat, and the hormone *thyroxin* does just that, plus regulates the metabolism. An under active thyroid can cause much unnecessary fat to be deposited all over the body. The lack of iodine, which occurs in consumption of over-refined food, is responsible for much thyroid trouble.

Mental sluggishness, difficulty in remembering, and the constant desire to sleep are typical problems of thyroid starvation. The thyroid has so many important functions in keeping people slim, trim and alert, in keeping the hair, nails and complexion healthy, that it could also be termed the "beauty master" of the body, reports Glayelord

Hauser. Not only can the wrong diet disturb the balance of this sensitive gland, but the resultant depression, fear, worry and constant strain can further weaken it.

Adequate iodine is of foremost importance for normal, healthy, functioning of the thyroid. Without it, people grow old before their time, lose their pep, become mentally lazy, lapsing into the blues, and never feeling warm enough (especially in the hands and feet).

"Dr. Russel Wilder of the Mayo Foundation has found that when human volunteers do not get sufficient vitamin B1, the thyroid gland becomes inactive, the basal metabolism drops far below normal, and the condition was not corrected by giving thyroid extract. It was corrected by giving Vitamin B1 without any thyroid. Probably thousands of people who now take thyroid extract would be helped far more by following a diet rich in all the B vitamins.

"Here then are the essential foods for a well balanced, smoothly functioning thyroid. First class proteins: low-fat meat, eggs...Abundant iodine: Shrimps, oysters, salmon, radishes, tomatoes, watercress, sea greens, cod liver oil and iodized vegetable salt. All the B vitamins, which are contained in brewer's yeast, yogurt, wheat germ and blackstrap molasses." [8]

Your *skin* is the largest organ of the body. If you were to stretch it out, it would cover about 18 square feet. That means there are many skin cells that have to be maintained and replaced. Most people think of the skin as being a passive organ, but it is very busy.

Let's look closer at the *skin's* needs.

Vitamin A

Vitamin A is essential for healthy skin and hair. A deficiency can cause your skin to react badly. Cells on the surface and even on several lower levels will shrivel up and die; the dead tissue will plug pores and all sacs. This results in whiteheads and blackheads, plus skin that resembles small goose pimples. In addition, without enough vitamin A, the skin becomes dry and rough.

Protein

Smooth, firm skin depends on good quality protein. Protein firms and tightens the skin because it comprises much of the elastic fiber that gives skin its tautness. Your best sources for improvement in firmness is protein, along with vitamins C and B complex. Protein is vital for good skin because skin is protein. It is a protein called keratin.

B complex

B complex nourishes the skin from the inside. It soothes away tension lines and helps regulate the thyroid gland for smooth, luminous skin. Daily stress can play havoc with your skin, and B vitamins are known to be morale boosters that help you handle stress better.

EPA (Omega-3 fatty acids)
"This is an excellent way to improve dry skin and to delay wrinkles. Cold water fish contain different kinds of fatty acids than those found in the usual American diet. These fatty acids have long names, such as elcosapentaenoic acid and docosahexaoic acid or EPA and DHA for short. These fatty acids are better for your skin than the types we usually consume. EPA is the best, but a good supplement will also contain DHA for balance.

"Reduce the total fat in your diet to about 25 percent of the calories. Then eat cold water fish such as sardines, haddock, tuna and salmon. Also, it is best to use olive oil." [8]

Vitamin E
Early aging can be prevented by taking Vitamin E, which is a free radical scavenger. It can significantly reduce the rate at which brown spots on the hand and other damage occurs.

Vitamin C
Vitamin C is essential to form a cementing substance called collagen. Dr. Bruce B Miller says, "Imagine your skin cells as protein bricks; the cement that holds these bricks in place is collagen. Without adequate cement (collagen), substances could leak

through the bricks (skin cells). In bruising, blood actually seeps through the poor collagen between the cells.

"Vitamin C is also essential for a normal, functioning thyroid. Your thyroid must be in good condition for smooth, porcelain-like skin.

"Vitamin C is a free radical scavenger much like vitamin E. The two actually work together, each working in a different area to protect your cells. Vitamin E is fat soluble and works best in the fatty areas of the cells, while Vitamin C is water soluble and works best in the watery areas of the cells.

"For skin, it is best to not take plain ascorbic acid only. Your supplement should contain 'C' plus nutrients called bioflavinoids which come with vitamin C in nature. The bioflavinoids will help maintain the integrity of the tiniest as well as the medium and small sized blood vessels." [10]

Herbal Laxative

Skin specialist, Dr. Bruce Miller, also writes, "The skin is the largest excretory organ in the body. With the number of toxins in our bodies to be excreted, our skin sometimes becomes excessively oily or blemished. This can result in pimples and other skin eruptions. To help relieve the skin of this excretory burden, I recommend the occasional use of a natural herbal laxative. Herbs have been used since the dawn of civilization to get things moving along more rapidly." [11]

HAIR

Hair grows from a tube which extends from near the surface of the epidermis deep into the dermis. This tube is called the hair follicle. Each follicle has its own oil producing gland, the sebaceous gland. The hair follicle bulges out at the bottom into the hair root. The hair grows from this root. As cells are added to the hair at the root, the hair is pushed up through the lubricated passage and eventually appears on the skin surface. (There are approximately 100,000 hairs on a human head.)

Let us look closer at the needed nutrients for hair health.

Protein

Your hair is at least 97 percent protein containing 19 of the 22 amino acids that form protein. If you are low in protein, you can expect your hair to reflect poor nutrition through breaking, cracking, and splitting. Also dryness, brittleness, and lack of luster along with hair loss may be signs of poor protein supplies. Because protein is not stored in the body for long, it should be replenished daily.

EPA

Same as for skin: You should try to take a supplement around 500 mg of EPA daily for best results. The Omega-3 fatty acids, DHA and EPA, are naturally found in fish, sea vegetables and eggs.

B complex for strong, evenly colored hair

The B complex, which are called as a group the "beauty vitamins" helps the hair in four distinct ways. Dr.Bruce Miller, who studied nutrition and also biochemistry, explains them as follows:

1. The complex is intimately involved in the formation and maintenance of a healthy hair shaft.
2. It smoothes the hair growth to an even, not jerky, rate of development.
3. Adequate B complex strengthens the hair shaft, so hair is strong and doesn't break easily.
4. It helps maintain consistent hair color. It is also mentioned in numerous studies as delaying the onset of graying hair; in a few cases it actually reversed some graying.

Zinc

Zinc is a mineral involved in areas of very rapid cell growth. Optimum nutrition, leading to faster hair growth, requires adequate amounts of zinc. Zinc can greatly strengthen the hair shaft by thickening it, resulting in full, luxurious hair.

Beta Carotene

See page 91. This nutrient improves hair and skin color and especially the sheen of your hair.

Special Note: The biggest destroyer of the B complex and zinc is stress. It is not enough to feed the body with proper nutrition and supplements, but it is important to learn how to deal with stress positively. All good foods and vitamin effect your hair and skin; the above mentioned are the basic essentials to good health.

Chapter 7

Antioxidants and the Immune System

Drs. Walter Pierpaoli and William Regelson state in their book, *The Melatonin Miracle,* that,"The immune system is actually a highly complex army of cells that protect the body against viruses, bacteria, and other foreign invaders, including some forms of cancer cells." [1]

The human immune system is broken down into cellular components called T helper cells and white blood cells that attack invading micro-organisms and humoral components, like antibodies and interferon that circulate in the body's fluids.

Brian Leibovitz, Ph.D., nutritional researcher at the University of California at Davis says, "When a white blood cell encounters an invading microbe, the uptake of oxygen increases by a factor of 30. At infectious sites, you get an abundance of the oxygen radicals formed and you need a dietary anti-oxidant to help protect the white blood cells."

According to recent studies, the following nutrients with anti-oxidant properties show promise in stimulating and protecting cellular immunity:

Vitamin A, Selenium, and Vitamin E.
Important in both cancer and immune therapy, Vitamin A makes the surface proteins of cancer cells more recognizable to the immune response system. Vitamin E can help control inflammations, and like selenium, is a powerful anti-oxidant against free radicals, which can stimulate cellular immunity.

Beta-Carotene, Zinc, and Vitamin B-6
Recent studies in *Immunology Letters* and the *American Journal of Clinical Nutrition* indicate that beta-carotene, zinc, and vitamin B6 can help enhance T helper cell lymphocytes that help identify and destroy invading organisms.

Beta carotene has been called "first among equals" by Arnold Fox, M.D., a regular contributor to *Let's Live.* He names it the single most important nutrient for the immune system. This is because beta-carotene is the body's vitamin A storage system.

Vitamin C and Bioflavonoids.

According to a study published by Ben Siegal, Ph.D., in *Infection and Immunity*, vitamin C may enhance interferon production and prevent viral infections. It also enhances the ability of a white blood cell to combat infections in bodily fluids. In a report in the *Proceedings of the American Association for Cancer Research,* bioflavonoids have been shown to inhibit reverse transcriptase, which takes viral RNA and makes it into DNA to infect human cells.

Vitamin C seems to play a role at almost every stage of immune function. It actually works inside the fighting cells where it helps convert glucose to energy, stimulates movement to the site of an infection, makes invading viruses and bacteria more susceptible to attack and makes them more receptive to chemical stimulation by other parts of the immune system.

In addition, vitamin C is an antioxidant and free radical scavenger. If sufficient vitamin C is circulating in the blood and tissues, it can scavenge the oxygen radicals which form as a by-product of the body's fight against any disease invasion and keep them from harming healthy cells.

Drs. Cheraskin, Ringsdorf, and Sisley explain the connection between vitamin C and the immune system in their book, *The Vitamin C Connection.* They show how white blood cells cruise about the body looking for "foreign enemies" to destroy. When white blood cells get sick, we get sick. The question was raised if vitamin C could help reduce abnormally high white-blood-cell counts that accompany many serious disorders. They did a test of 1,043 people. The results were this: "In short vitamin C can help when there are too few white blood cells and when there are too many." [2]

Pycnogenols

Pycnogenols (pronounced pick-nah' geh-nols) are standardized extracts of either pine bark or grape seed. Chemically they are known as PCOs, a type of bioflavonoid. PCOs have been found to be incredible antioxidants (cell protectors). Testing shows PCOs to be 50 times more potent than vitamin E as an antioxidant and 20 more potent than vitamin C. Dr. Rothchild, a 1986 Nobel Prize nominee and pioneer PCO researcher, explains its value: "It's the only barrier, providing extra protection from the free radical damage throughout the nervous system."

In general, PCOs are known to have a number of beneficial activities. They have a strengthening effect on the capillaries. This makes them important in helping to treat diabetic retinopathy, heart disease, varicose veins, bruising and other peripheral vascular disorders.

Omega-3 Fatty Acids and Glutathione

Data published in the *Journal of Nutrition* suggests that omega-3 fatty acids may stimulate the T lymphocytes in the immune system. The anti-oxidant glutathione may help detoxify drugs which cause side effects in the immune compromised patient.

Protein

Many functions of the immune system depend on adequate protein intake. Although individual needs vary, the RDA is 45-65 grams daily. Make sure to get sufficient protein especially when dieting or fighting illness or infection. If there is not sufficient protein available, the body will take it from muscle tissue, among other places.

While the body fights disease, it burns amino acids that it metabolizes from protein. During an infection, the lifespan of white blood cells is greatly shortened. Cells which normally live four to five days may need to be replaced after only a few hours. Amino acids can slow the breakdown, keeping the infection fighting cells active.

Garlic and Germanium

Garlic is not only anti-fungal, but it is an immuno-stimulatory agent according to a study published in the *Journal of Immunology*. The metabolic energy enhancer, germanium, has also been shown to induce the synthesis of interferon from the white blood cells, and may have an emerging role in the treatment of many diseases, according to Jeffrey Reinhard, M.S., a nutritional biochemist with the

Marin Clinic of Preventive Medicine and Health Education.

Immune Enhancing Herbs

The Chinese government has poured millions of dollars into research on herbs that traditional Chinese doctors had claimed would protect and bolster the immune system. Though several have been listed in various studies, three stand out in their ability to enhance phagocytosis, promote lymphocytic transformation, restore blood cell production, and increase cellular immunity: Ginseng, Astragalus, and Skiitake.

Echinacea has been called "the most effective and accessible immune enhancing herb available today." Echinacea contains compounds found to be antibacterial and antiviral.

Positive Thinking

New studies have proven that the mind and immune system are strongly linked. What happens in the mind invariably affects the immune system. In the book, *Anatomy of an Illness,* Norman Cousins shares his quest for health when he contacted a disease of the connective tissue. He was told that there was no cure.

He decided to talk to his doctor about some things he thought would help him get better. First, he considered the medication. The hospital had been giving him massive doses. He thought it was unreasonable to expect positive chemical changes to take place so long as his body was being saturated with pain-killing medications. He asked his doctor, Dr. Hitzig, if he could start having injections of ascorbic acid (Vitamin C). He had read that vitamin C helps to oxygenate the blood, and that people suffering from collagen diseases are deficient in vitamin C. He also changed his diet to include only fresh vegetables, fruits and foods high in nutrients.

Secondly, he writes, "I knew that pain could be affected by attitudes." He had the nurse bring films that were funny and made him laugh. He said, "It worked. I made the joyous discovery that ten minutes of genuine belly laughter had an anesthetic effect and would give me at least two hours of pain-free sleep...How scientific was it to believe that laughter—as well as the positive emotions in general—was affecting my body chemistry for the better?...was greatly elated by the discovery that there is a physiologic basis for the ancient theory that laughter is good medicine." [3]

Exercise

Exercise works on both the physical and psychological levels; improving health and increasing resistance to disease. It is an excellent immune builder. Studies suggest that the natural pain-killers produced by the brain during a strenuous workout can increase immune system activity. Endorphins enhance the activity of T-cells and other killer cells.

Exercise also stimulates the growth of the thymus gland (where lymphocytes taken from the blood stream are trained to function as T-cells).

Elevated body temperature produced by exercise has also been shown to boost immune activity, and exercise has enhanced the effects of vitamins A and C. In addition, the activity of interferon doubled in otherwise inactive individuals after an hour of steady exercise.

Special Note: Overconsumption of some foods can inhibit the immune function. These foods are mainly sugar and fat. Siri Khalsa reports in *Nutrition News,* 1988, Vol. XI, No. 1 that, "One hundred gram portions of simple carbohydrate (25 teaspoons of crystals, a little more than the sugar in two sodas) can significantly decrease the ability of certain white blood cells to devour harmful substances in the body (neutrophil phagocytic activity) for up to five hours and longer, and can also decrease the transformation of other white blood cells (lymphocytes) into T-cells.

"A diet high in saturated fats may suppress some functions of the immune system by interfering with the production of prostaglandin E1."

Summary: Sleep and exercise have notable effects on susceptibility to disease. They can relieve stress and support proper circulation, excretion, and metabolism. They also have a stimulating effect on interleukin and interferon production and activity.

Proper nutrition, cleanliness, adequate rest and recreation, regular exercise and a positive outlook on life are keys to good health and ways to enhance the immune system.

Jean Won reports in "The Walking Magazine," in the January/February issue, that Mohsen Meydani, Ph.D., an associate professor of nutrition at Tufts University, says that antioxidants-namely beta carotene and Vitamin C and E-are nutrients that fight heart diesease and certain cancers. Beta carotene and vitamin C are effective in preventing cancer-causing cells from multiplying, he says. Jean Won names carrots, citrus fruits, and any orange-yellow squash as being good sources of vitamin C and beta carotene. Vitamin E is found mainly in vegetable oils, nuts, and seeds.

Chapter 8

A Healthy Colon

The small intestine is twenty-two feet long, and is where digestion is completed and all absorption of nutrients occurs. It has an alkaline environment, brought about by highly alkaline bile, pancreatic juice, and secretions of the intestinal walls. The three parts of the small intestine are the following: the first part, the *duodenum*, which begins at the stomach outlet, the second part, the *jejunum* (about ten feet long), and the third part, the *ileum*, which is ten to twelve feet long. Any material leaving the ileum and entering the cecum (where the small and large intestines join) is quite watery. Backflow is prevented at this junction by a muscular valve. Very little is absorbed from the large intestine except water.

The large intestine is known as the *colon*. The colon is primarily a storage and dehydrating organ. Substances entering in a liquid state become semisolid as water is absorbed. It takes twelve to fourteen hours for contents to make the circuit of the intestine. The colon is populated with bacteria, normal intestinal flora. A large part of the feces is composed of bacteria, along with indigestible material, chiefly cellulose, and substances eliminated from the blood and the intestinal walls.

The colon and bowel are the depository for all waste material after food nutrients have been extracted and processed to the bloodstream. Decaying food ferments, forms gases, as well as toxins, and the colon becomes a breeding ground for putrefactive bacteria, viruses, parasites, yeasts, molds, etc. Ideally, one should eliminate as often as a meal is taken in. Bowel transit time should be approximately 12 hours. To promote healthy bowel function, include plenty of fiber and liquids in your diet, exercise regularly and establish a regular time for elimination.

Good colon health foods are flax seed, bran, brewer's yeast, yogurt, acidolphilus, greens. A low fat diet, with plenty of high fiber fruits, whole grains, cereals, salad greens, and cultured foods like yogurt and kefir to establish friendly intestinal flora are necessary for good elimination. It is important to avoid all refined foods, saturated fats, fried food, and caffeine. It is essential to drink 6-8 glasses of water a day.

Aloe vera is one of the finest internal body cleansers. It cleans diseased or unwanted matter from the stomach, liver, kidneys, spleen and bladder. Many feel it is the finest colon cleaner in existence. It is healing and soothing to the stomach, a superlative digestive aid, plus giving relief from stomach distress and ulcers. For these kinds of problems, a pint of Aloe vera juice or gel should be taken each day on an empty stomach. Also aloe pills can act as a natural laxative and purifier. (We use *Aloelax*, which is a herbal stimulant laxative, made by "Nature's Way").

Several years ago the subject of alimentary toxemia was discussed in London before the Royal Society of Medicine, fifty-seven of the leading physicians of Great Britain. Among the speakers were eminent surgeons, physicians, and specialists in the various branches of medicine. They discussed 36 highly active poisons. In cases of alimentary toxemia some one or several of these poisons is constantly bathing the delicate body cells, which finally result in grave disease. The digestive organs, heart and blood vessels, the nervous system, the eyes, and the skin are all affected by the health of the colon.

The physicians mentioned above concluded that the following diseases could eventually be the outcome of alimentary toxemia. The title of the article was, "Death Begins in the Colon." The article stated, "It should be understood that these findings are not mere theories, but are the results of demonstration in actual practice by eminent physicians. Of course, it is not claimed that alimentary toxemia is the only cause of all the symptoms and diseases named: although of many it may be the sole or principal cause, some of them are due to other causes as well. In the following summary the various symptoms and disorders mentioned in the discussion in London are grouped and classified."

The Digestive Organs
Duodenal ulcer causing partial or complete obstruction of the duodenum
Pyloric spasm
Pyloric obstruction
Distention and dilation of the stomach
Gastric ulcer
Cancer of the stomach
Inflammation of the liver
Cancer of the liver
Foul gases and foul smelling stools
Colitis
Appendicitis, acute and chronic
Inflammation of pancreas
Enlargement of spleen
Cancer of pancreas
Inflammatory changes of gall bladder
Cancer of gall bladder

Gallstones
Degeneration of liver
Infection of the gums and decay of the teeth
Ulcers in the mouth and pharynx

Heart and Blood Vessels
Wasting and weakening of the heart muscles
Fatty degeneration of the heart
Endocarditis
Subnormal blood pressure
Enlargement of the heart
The dilatation of the aorta
High blood pressure
Arteriosclerosis
Permanent dilation of arteries
Dr. W. Berley says, "There are a few phases of cardiovascular trouble (disease of heart and blood vessels) with which disorder of some part of the alimentary tract is not causatively associated."

The Nervous System
Headaches of various kinds: frontal, occipital, temporal, dull or intense, hemicrania
Headache of a character that leads to a mistaken diagnosis of brain tumor.
(Dr. Lane tells of a case where a surgeon had proposed an operation for the removal of a tumor from the frontal lobe of the brain; the difficulty was wholly removed by the exclusion of the colon.)
Acute neuralgia pains in the legs

Neuritis
Twitching of the eyes and of muscles of face, arms, legs, etc.
Lassitude
Irritability
Disturbance of nervous system, varying from simple headaches to absolute collapse
Mental and physical depression
Insomnia
Troubled sleep
Unpleasant dreams
The patient awakening tired
Excessive sleepiness
Fatigue
Difficulty of mental concentration

The Eyes
Degenerative changes in the eye
Inflammation of the lens
Inflammation of the optic nerve
Hardening of lens
Sclerotitis
Iritis
Cataract
Recurrent hemorrhage in the retina
Eye dull and heavy

The Skin
Formation of wrinkles
Thin, inelastic, starchy skin

Pigmentations of the skin: yellow, brown, blue, muddy complexion
Thickening of the skin
Boils and sores
Eczema
Dermatitis
Lupus erythemarosus
Acne rosacrea
Dark circles under the eyes
Psoriasis
Pityriasis
Jaundice
"An infinitesimal amount of poison may suffice to cause skin eruption."

It is also understood that stress can adversely affect the colon, and just as important as foods are to the body and in keeping the colon clean from toxins, the condition of the nerves and the way one handles stress is significant also. However, it is *essential* to keep the colon clean from toxic matter if you want a healthy body.

Chapter 9

Menopause With a Smile

As the years slip by, the body changes gradually, and needs extra help in order to retain good health. Somewhere around age 40 or 50, things start to change in a woman's body, and the process of menopause begins (the termination of the reproductive period in a female). This time of your life should be one of the happiest times ever, and it can be if you stay well-informed and discipline yourself to a healthy lifestyle.

Calcium: According to Lawrence Lamb, M.D., a well-known syndicated columnist, this vulnerable period is one fact that causes women of age sixty or over to have osteoporosis. Although the need for calcium is a must for all adults, women especially need extra intake when entering menopause.

Good calcium foods are sardines, salmon, dark leafy greens and broccoli. It is also good to take a Cal-Mag supplement daily.

Vitamin D aids the absorption of calcium, helps its retention, and improves its utilization. Adelle Davis writes, "This vitamin is particularly needed during the menopause, when the calcium intake is usually low. Hot flashes, night sweats, leg cramps, irritability, nervousness, and mental depression, so frequently experienced at this time, can be overcome in a single day by giving calcium and vitamin D.

"During the menopause, the lack of ovarian hormones causes severe calcium-deficiency symptoms to occur; at these time unusually large amounts of calcium should be obtained and every step be taken to insure its absorption into the blood." [1]

Boron: Researchers for the U.S. Department of Agriculture have recently found that boron helps to prevent osteoporosis. Twelve women given modest boron supplements (3 mg. a day) showed significantly reduced losses of calcium, magnesium and phosphorus, indicating that these minerals were not being lost from bone tissue. Plant foods like apples, pears, and broccoli are rich in boron; meat and fish are not.

Vitamin E: Extra vitamin E is also needed at this time of a woman's life. A lack of vitamin E reveals itself in the form of brown ceroid pigment which remains whenever unsaturated fatty acids are destroyed by oxygen. Adelle Davis writes, "I suspect the ugly brown spots on the backs of hands of persons middle-aged or older result from a vitamin E deficiency; they usually appear at menopause, when the vitamin requirement skyrockets, especially when female hormones are taken which increase the vitamin E need tenfold.

"Cumulative menstrual losses, pregnancies, and the long use of deficient diets cause anemia to be prevalent in women at and after the menopause. Besides causing needless fatigue, mental confusion, and depression, anemia can bring about such forgetfulness that these women often become convinced they are losing their minds." [2]

Iron and Iodine: Not only is extra iron needed by the body but also iodine. Adelle Davis writes, "The iodine requirements are increased in early childhood, puberty, and adolescence, during pregnancy and lactation, and particularly at menopause. It is during menopause that goiters most often grow to be huge . . . Before the thyroid glands can become normal again, an adequate diet supplemented daily with both iodine and vitamin E must be maintained for many months. Even large goiters can, however, often disappear in time . . . Additional amounts of iodine appear not to be needed at these times *if* iodized salt has been used continuously for years; the thyroid gland traps and stores iodine for future safety."

It would be a good thing to eat foods that contained calcium, vitamins D and E, iron, and iodine, and since anemia is related to a lack of certain B vitamins, it would also be beneficial to include foods that contained them.

Tyrosine: Studies by Dr. Alan Gelenberg at Harvard University found tyrosine to be extremely effective for depression, even in patients that would not respond to conventional antidepressant therapy. This can be purchased at any health store.

Dr. Murray, heard on *Healthline*, during a KCJH radio interview, discussed a product called FemTrol, which is strictly for women, especially those who are in menopause. His mother started taking it, then got all her friends to take it, and they all were enthusiastic reporting excellent results. The herbs listed on the bottle include Black Cohash Extract, Dong Quai Extract, Licorice Root Extract, Chaste Berry Extract, False Unicorn Root Extract and Fennel Seed Extract.

Black Cohash acts as a female estrogen. It helps relieve menstrual cramps, high blood pressure, and hot flashes. It calms the nervous system and relieves tension.

Dong Quai is high in B12 and helps relieve hot flashes, migraines, nourishes the blood and relaxes the muscles.

Licorice Root helps hypoglycemia, adrenal glands, stress, voice and colds. It helps the body make cortisone.

Chaste Berry (Vitex agnus-castus) is becoming widely used as an herb that addresses various hormonal imbalances in women. The effects of Vitex are thought to be due to some regulatory effect upon the pituitary gland. Recent findings confirm that chasteberry helps restore a normal estrogen-to-progesterone balance. It is especially beneficial during menopausal changes, relieving symptoms such as hot flashes, and emotional changes. It is available in capsule or liquid form.

Herbalist Lesley Tierra, states in her book, *The Herbs of Life*, "Chasteberry, also referred to as vitex, is a supreme Female herb. It stimulates the pituitary gland and the secretion of luteotropic hormone which increases the output of progesterone. Thus, it regulates hormonal balance and the menstrual cycle, including normalizing estrogen . . . It also aids problems associated with menopause such as dry vagina, hot flashes, dizziness and depression." [3]

False Unicorn and *Fennel Seed* also help ease menopause.

Other herbs, oils and such that are known to help women during menopause are as follows:

Damiana is known as a lady's aphrodisiac. It helps the body make female hormones. Damiana is primarily used for treating female problems in Mexico. It is excellent at restoring an exhausted state of the body and increasing its vital energies. For women, it has been found to strengthen reproductive organs and helps with menopause, by controlling and reducing hot flashes. It has also been used to strengthen the ovum in the female and it also helps to balance the hormones in woman.

Passion Flower helps ease menopause, headaches, hysteria or hypertension.

Feverfew (tanacetum parthenium) is an herbal remedy that dates back to Greco-Roman times. It helps relieve most migraines at onset. It helps PMS, menopause, stress, hay fever and psoriasis.

Evening Primrose Oil contains GLA (Gamma Linoleic Acid). It is a source of energy for the cells, electrical insulation for nerve fibers, and helps regulates hormone and metabolic functions. Therapeutic use is wide ranging from control of PMS and menopause symptoms, to help in nerve transmission for M.S. and muscular dystrophy.

There is an excellent product that works quite well when taken at bedtime to alleviate night sweats, insomnia, etc. It is called *Ultra-Cal Night* by "Source Naturals." It contains Calcium, Magnesium, Maganese, Boron, Silicon, Copper, vitamin B6, vitamin C, vitamin D3, L-Glutamic Acid, L-Lysine, and Herbal formula consisting of Horsetail Silica extract, Alfalfa leaf, Nettles, Yellow Dock & Dulse.

In the book, *The Melatonin Miracle,* Drs. Walter Pierpaoli and William Regelson recommend taking Melatonin during the menopausal years. Melatonin, they say, is nature's age-reversing, disease-fighting, sex-enhancing hormone. It is a hormone produced by the body in the pineal gland, a pea-sized structure embedded within the brain, and is the key to understanding, and controlling, how we age. As we age, our melatonin levels start to decrease.

It is not unusual for a menopausal woman to be abruptly awakened by a hot flash, or to suffer from insomnia. Drs. Pierpaoli and Regelson say, "The fact that older people and menopausal women are plagued by sleep problems is no coincidence. In both cases, melatonin levels have started their decline, and the disruption in melatonin cycling makes getting a good night's sleep difficult...Melatonin supplements can normalize sleep patterns, and sleeping well is absolutely critical to a restorative and rejuvenating rest." [4]

In my research, I came across DHEA. Health counselor, Siri Khalsa, reports in *Nutrition News*, 1996, Vol. XX, No. 2, the following information: "For over a decade, the DHEA phyto-precursors provided in wild yam have been providing women with an alternative to synthetic hormones. Wild yam has been especially recommended for 'women's problems,' specifically PMS and menopausal symptoms. The work of both John R. Lee, M.D. and Raymond Peat, Ph.D, in promoting this natural therapy has improved the lives of hundreds of thousands of women." For more information concerning this necessary hormone in the body, consult a good health store. The supplement, DHEA, can also be purchased from them.

New research reveals also that soy foods can lower cholesterol, fight breast cancer, slow bone loss, and relieve side effects of menopause. Peter Jaret reports in the January, 1996 issue of "Hippocrates," a magazine of health and medicine for Physicians, the following information: "In one study at the University of Milan, patients who stuck to a moderately low-fat diet had only modest decreases in cholesterol, but when researchers added soy protein to their diets, without making any other changes, their 'bad' LDL cholesterol fell an average of 21 percent in three weeks...By comparing before-and-after bone scans, they'll also investigate whether soy foods can really retard osteoporosis as scientists suspect. Based on animal studies, the premise hinges on those estrogen look-alikes in soy. Called isoflavones, these bear so strong a resemblance to the hormone in a woman's body that they may be able to fill in when her own levels start to fall."

Jaret continues to report, "That's more than conjecture. At the Dunn Clinical Nutrition Centre, in Cambridge, England, researchers have shown that daily servings of soy protein lengthen menstrual cycles in premenopausal women, suggesting an estrogenlike effect. Also, several as-yet-unpublished studies suggest that isoflavones can alleviate hot flashes and night sweats in menopausal women, according to Mark Messina, a former program director in the Diet and Cancer branch of the National Cancer Institute who recently organized the first international symposium on soy foods and health. While more studies are needed, he's optimistic: 'I'd bet good money soy protein will become a widely accepted alternative to estrogen replacement therapy within the next few years.'

"Soy isn't the only source of plant estrogens; scientists have identified three different kinds that are found in hundreds of other foods, from carrots and potatoes to bean sprouts and sunflower seeds. Yet soy is a particularly rich source, and there's growing evidence that a particular *form* of isoflavone it contains could actually defend against cancer of many kinds. Called genistein, it's a potent antioxidant, able to snare unstable oxygen molecules before they turn healthy cells cancerous.

"Genistein also appears to block several key enzymes that tumor cells need to grow and thrive, and studies show it may also thwart the growth of blood vessels supplying those cells, effectively starving them at the source. The findings are so impressive that the National Cancer Institute is now studying the potential of purified genistein as an anticancer drug.

"'But why wait?' Messina says. Genistein is so abundant in soy foods that one serving a day, he suspects—a glass of soy milk, a half-cup of firm tofu, or a couple of those Breakfast Club muffins (these were muffins laced with generous portions of soy protein, served three times a week in the food science department at the University of Illinois in

Champaign-Urbana, conducted by food scientist, John Erdman, Jr.), is probably enough for most of us to substantially lessen our cancer risk.

"It's worth the trouble, if you ask study veteran Karen Hyde. When she started on soy, her total cholesterol stood at a hazardous 255; six months later it was 205. And as her LDL cholesterol went down, her HDL–the good kind–went up. 'My doctor could hardly believe it,' she says."

Author's Note: Many women have asked what herbs I take. Each morning upon arising, before eating breakfast, I take the following herb capsules, which I have found to be excellent and very helpful– (They really do work):

a. *Every Woman's Natural Health–Women's Phase II*
b. *Femtrol*
   (a & b contain many of the herbs discussed in this chapter.)
c. *Gink Alert–Ginkgo Biloba Special Formula*
d. *Ginseng Siberian Extract* 200 Extract
e. *Damiana Leaves*
f. *St. John's Wort*
g. *Gota Kola*
h. *Fo-Ti–Ho-Shou-Wa*
I. *Evening Primrose Oil*

Chapter 10

Ways to Fight Cancer

Although cancer is not completely understood, there are theories that indicate that emotions, beliefs and attitudes, as well as poor diet, can cause cancer cells to increase. Dr. Bernie S. Siegel suggests that cancer cells can become more prominent when the tension and anxiety of modern life keep the stress response "on" continually. He writes, "The immune system, is controlled by the brain, either indirectly through hormones in the bloodstream, or directly through the nerves and neurochemicals. One of the most widely accepted explanations of cancer, the 'surveillance' theory, states that cancer cells are developing in our bodies all the time but are normally destroyed by white blood cells before they can develop into dangerous tumors. Cancer appears when the immune system becomes suppressed and can no longer deal with this routine threat. It follows that whatever upsets the brain's control of the immune system will foster malignancy." [1]

Throughout this book, the things that will help fight against cancer is alluded to quite frequently, though at times in an unobstrusive manner. This chapter will simply enlarge upon several of those vital nutrients that possibly have already been mentioned. It is a conclusive fact that diet does affect a person's health. The *FDA Consumer,* April, 1988, reported that 80 percent of cancers may be related to the way people live, whether they smoke and what they eat, for example, rather than to forces beyond their control. Let us look at several nutrients that have been studied, researched, tested, and concluded by many to have important nutrients to help combat cancer.

Selenium

"Dr. Larry Clark of Cornell University, Ithaca, N.Y., found that people with low blood selenium levels had four times the skin cancer rate as those with high levels. He also researched more serious kinds of cancer in relation to blood levels of selenium and discovered that patients in the lowest one-tenth of the population in terms of blood selenium levels showed six times the incidence of cancer as those in the highest one-tenth of the population.

"Gerhard Schrauzer, Ph.D., found that selenium supplements help to guard against breast cancer. Research projects demonstrate that selenium is even more effective as insurance against cancer when teamed with vitamin E." [2]

Sources of Selenium
*Brazil nuts
Brown rice   Garlic
Wheat germ   Whole Grains
Onions   Molasses
Brewers Yeast   Salmon

*Holly McCord, RD says in Prevention magazine, "The richest source of selenium with 30 times more than any other food is the brazil nut! It takes only one or two to get the entire daily Recommended Dietary Allowance for selenium. But if you're nuts about Brazil nuts, beware: They're so stuffed with selenium that eating too many on a regular basis-a big handful every day-could lead to selenium toxicity. On the other hand, a Brazil nut or two a day on top of a normal diet is reasonable. Selenium acts in our bodies as a key player against unstable molecules that may cause cancer and heart disease." [3]

Vitamin C
In 1966, Dr. Ewan Cameron, chief surgeon of the Vale of Leven Hospital, Loch Lomondside,

Scotland, published his thesis that the most important determinant in the incidence, progress, and outcome of cancer is the body's own protective mechanisms, and that considerable control over cancer might be achieved if some way could be found to enhance these natural defenses. Dr. Linus Pauling contacted Dr. Cameron espousing the use of vitamin C for this purpose. He gives this account of Dr. Cameron's response: "...his immediate reaction to the idea that vitamin C could have value against cancer was sheer incredulity. He has said that he was a conservative Scottish surgeon, and that the people around him... were conservative Scottish medical people. It seemed quite ludicrous to them to suggest that this simple, cheap, harmless powder, which could be bought in any drugstore, could possibly have any value against such a bafflingly complex and resistant disease as cancer."

The result of Dr. Cameron's encounter with Dr. Pauling is now history. Dr. Pauling prevailed and Dr. Cameron went along with him, deciding to make use of vitamin C in a trial using 100 patients with advanced cancer. These patients were treated with 10 grams of C per day, both orally and intravenously. The results of their progress was matched against the records of 1000 other cancer patients. These 1000 controls were matched to the 100 vitamin C patients by age, sex, and primary tumor type. All 1100 subjects were diagnosed as having terminal cancer. At the end of a year, 22 of the 100 patients survived while only 4 of the 1000 controls lived more than a year. In an interview with *Bestways* (1978), Dr. Pauling stated that the patients were still living after seven years, while all of the controls had died.

Dr. Cameron was particularly gratified by the positive side effects experienced by his patients. He said instead of feeling miserable, they became lively, regained appetite, and often were able to go home and return to work. He also discovered that vitamin C worked so effectively as a pain killer that he was able to stop administering opiates.

Siri Khalsa reports in *Nutrition News* that, "Cancer itself is not a significant disease caused by one agent. Cancer specialists have defined five basic cancers and within these divisions there are at least 200 different types...All of these cancers have some mutual characteristics, one of which is the basic condition of cancer itself. This is a condition in which previously normal cells from any tissue in the body suffer a change that makes them grow and reproduce in an uncontrolled fashion."

It is very interesting to note that "88 percent of all cancers originate from organs that contain less than 4.5 mg of vitamin C per 100 grams of organ tissue. Only 12 percent of cancers originate from organs containing higher concentrations." [4]

Tomatoes

Holly McCord, RD says in *Prevention* magazine, "To help keep doctors away, eat something tomato every day! Scientists found recently that people in northern Italy who ate seven or more servings of raw tomatoes every week had 60 percent less chance of developing colon, rectal and stomach cancer than people who ate only two servings or less (International Journal of Cancer, October 14, 1994).

"What's so plummy about tomatoes? According to Dr. Colditz, tomatoes are one of the few foods rich in an antioxidant called lycopene, a member of the carotenoid clan, that's been overshadowed till now by its famous cousin, beta-carotene. Scientists think antioxidants from veggies and fruit become commandos against cancer inside our bodies. (Besides lycopene, tomatoes have vitamin C and p-coumaric and chlorogenic acids, even *more* antioxidants!)." [5]

The January, 1996 issue of *Health Counselor*, agrees with this. They did an essay on the article "Eat Smart," by Jean Carper, a health columnist for the "USA Weekend" newspaper, printed September 1995. She wrote that tomatoes have an active compound that is twice as potent as beta carotene. Tomatoes contain lycopenes which, in laboratory tests, have been shown to be extremely effective at killing free radicals, which promote aging and many chronic illnesses.

Carper explained that Italian researchers found that people who ate the most raw tomatoes had only one half the risk of developing digestive tract cancers. John Hopkins researchers also discovered in a study of 26,000 people that those with the lowest levels of lycopenes in their blood had a five times greater chance of developing pancreatic cancer than those with high levels of lycopenes.

"Lycopenes are not destroyed by heat and are in every tomato product. They are strong antioxidants that help protect healthy cells. Two medium ripe tomatoes, one cup of canned tomatoes, two tablespoons of tomato paste, one-half cup tomato sauce, three-fourths cup of tomato soup, and three-fourths cup tomato juice, all contain 20 mg. of lycopenes. It is not known yet how much lycopene is necessary for optimum health."

Fruits and Green and Yellow Vegetables

The 1992 summer issue of the magazine *Health News,* included the following information in the article entitled "How the carrot locks up free radicals:"

For years, scientists have noticed that people who eat lots of green and yellow vegetables have a lower incidence of cataracts or lung cancer...Biomedical researchers suspect a common byproduct of chemical reaction in the body–called free radicals–may lead to diseases as diverse as cancer or cataracts. They are also investigating how other molecules may protect the body from free radical damage.

Every chemical or compound has an overwhelming longing to be neutral-neither positive nor negative. Free radicals are charged molecules, meaning they are hungry for an electron or two. Starving is more like it. Their desire to have a neutral charge is so compelling that they are likely to rob an electron from any nearby molecule to satisfy their appetite. To the free radical, it makes no difference whether it robs DNA, a lipid in a cell wall, or simply a stray H20. It will do what it must to get another electron.

But for the attacked molecule, the consequences may be fatal. Free radicals can damage the micro-building blocks of cell walls, weakening the cell. Giant molecules of DNA can be broken apart and thus lose their ability to guide healthy cell life.

There is a natural defense against free radicals: vitamins and minerals. The body's enzymes use minerals like selenium, copper, zinc, and manganese (antioxidants) to capture and neutralize free radicals.

Vitamins from leafy yellow and green vegetables like carrots are large molecules which float around the body soaking up free radicals like sponges before they attack other molecules. So eat your vegetables.

So now you know why your mother and father always said, "Eat your vegetables." They may not have understood why, but they were right on track.

Peter Greenwald, Ph.D., director of the division of cancer prevention and control at the National Cancer Institute has stated, "Right now, we know of over 1,000 chemical compounds, many of them found naturally in vegetables, that have the potential to inhibit cancer development."

Vegetables are important in cancer prevention, but fruits are also important. Research scientists have found that grapes and strawberries contain ellagic acid, which binds some chemical carcinogens and may be effective in preventing the development of colon or esophageal cancer. A natural flavoring agent that's present in oranges and lemons and known as d-limonene is also being studied for its potential use, in a purified form, as a chemopreventer.

Diane S. Klein writes in the July, 1994 issue of the *Ladies Home Journal,* on the subject, "The Anti-Breast Cancer." She lists the top ten vegetables reprinted from *How to Reduce Your Risk of Breast Cancer,* written by Jon F. Mihovicz, M.D., Ph.D., who is on staff at Rockefeller University, in New York City, and is the director and founder of the Foundation for Preventive Oncology. They are the following:

Broccoli,
Brussels sprouts,
Cabbage,
Cauliflower,
Collards,
Kale,
Radishes,
Rutabaga,
Turnip
Watercress.

    Ms. Klein summarizes her article by saying, "Remember, eating healthful foods doesn't mean being stuck with a dull and boring diet. Try new recipes and experiment with new fruits and vegetables. Look for way to substitute the 'right' foods for ones that are high in fat. Before long, you'll become accustomed to these new tastes and will realize how enjoyable they can be. And, best of all, you will be taking a key step in lowering your risk of breast cancer.

    "Cancer researchers at the Massachusetts Institute of Technology have found that vitamins C and E and certain chemicals called *indoles*, found in cabbage, Brussels sprouts, and related vegetables in the crucifer family, are potent and apparently safe inhibitors of certain carcinogens." [6]

    Diane Hales reports the following in her article, "Cut Your Cancer Risk," in the February 1, 1995, *Woman's Day*, magazine. "Researches at the Johns Hopkins Medical Institutions have identified a cancer-blocking compound called *sulforaphane* in broccoli and other 'cruifers.'" In this same article, Marion Nestle, Ph.D., who heads the nutrition department at New York University, says, "Eating more fruits and vegetables is the number-one dietary guideline for lowering your cancer risk."

Beta-Carotene and Vitamin E

There is much discussion about the discovery of a link between cancer and carotene. Siri Khalsa, reports in *Nutrition News, 1989, Volume XII, No. 11,* that increased intake of fruits and vegetables, especially those rich in carotenes, appear to reduce the risk of epithelial cancers. These include cancer of the lung and stomach, and possibly of the ovaries, breast, cervix, prostate, larynx, tongue, mouth, esophagus, and bladder. (One cooked sweet potato contains 24,880 IU's of Vitamin A (carotene) and 1 cooked carrot contains 19,150 IU's. Eating these is one way to assimilate carotene into your body.)

"The evidence is very promising," says Gerald Sklar of Harvard. "Beta-carotene and vitamin E are the first nontoxic agents that can both prevent and reverse cancer in experimental animals."

In one study of lung cancer appearing in the *New England Journal of Medicine,* Menkes, et al. reported that subjects with vitamin E blood levels in the lowest fifth of the sample had a 2.5 times greater risk of lung cancer than subjects with the highest vitamin E blood levels (1986).

Concerning breast cancer, Wald, et al. analyzed blood samples from 39 women who later developed breast cancer with 78 matched controls and found that there was a clear association between plasma vitamin E levels and breast cancer risk. In this study, women with vitamin E levels in the lowest fifth of the sample had a breast cancer risk five times greater than women with vitamin E plasma levels in the highest fifth (*British Journal of Cancer*, 1984).

Garlic

Siri Khalsa, reports the following in *Nutrition News*, 1995, Vol. XIX, No. 11: "Possibly the greatest motivator for the scientific investigation of garlic in the U.S. has been the findings of population studies in China and in Italy. According to the data, there is an inverse relationship between garlic intake and cancer rates. People who eat the most garlic have the least cancer...garlic is much more effective than Vitamin C in blocking nitrosamine formation."

In *The New York Times'* "Science Times," Jane Brody summarized the effects of garlic against cancer, stating that it blocks the ability of carcinogens to transform normal cells into cancer as well as inhibiting the early growth of some transformed cells; that it stimulates various immunological factors that may helps the body to combat cancer; and that its antioxidant effect protects against damage by pollutants so ubiquitous in today's urban and industrial environments. In commenting on garlic and cancer, researcher Stephen Fulder writes, "This does not mean that garlic treats cancers. Rather, it helps to prevent them."

The average clove contains seven calories, vitamins B1, 2, and 3, and vitamin C, plus the minerals calcium, iron, potassium, phosphorus, selenium, manganese, zinc, germanium and copper. According to an article in *Natural Foods Merchandiser* it contains all eight essential amino acids and the highest sulfur content of all the vegetables.

Besides sulfur, garlic also contains the highest level of the mineral selenium of any plant. It is believed that this high level of biologically active selenium may account for garlic's anti-atherosclerotic property. Although selenium has long been recognized as necessary for livestock health, it was not until the late 70s that some researchers began to believe that selenium might also protect against human heart attack, stroke, hypertension and cancer.

Garlic is also one of the best natural sources of germanium. Dr. Kazuhiko Asai has devoted years of his life to germanium research and has hailed it as a miracle cure for everything from headaches to life threatening conditions.

Certain Herbs

In my research, I came across an unknown herb to me, *Pau D'Arco/Taheebo*. It is given free by the Argentina government to cancer and leukemia patients. It is known to discourage Candida Albicans, herpes simplex, anemia, pain, and reduces tumors/polyps, and strengthens the immune system.

Chaparral has also been know to dissolve tumors. It is a blood purifier and cleanser.

Echinacea/Parthenium is a blood and lymph cleaner, has mild antibiotic activity. Interferon-like, cortisone-like (anti-inflammatory), increases T-cells, demonstrates anti-tumor activity and stimulates the immune response.

Siberian ginseng does not kill cancer cells. Experiments have shown that it **reinforces antitumor immunity**, **retards the development of metastases** and increases the effects of chemo and radiation therapies while alleviating their side effects. In Chinese hospitals, it is used to protect the immune systems of cancer patients undergoing chemotherapy. In the USSR its use is highly recommended as an adjunct to any cancer treatment.

Soviet observations have shown that when Siberian ginseng was taken two to four days prior to the beginning of treatment or simultaneously with it, the patients showed almost none of the usual reactions such as indisposition, dizziness, nausea, loss of appetite, etc.

The following interviews with three different Doctors substantiates that food and nutrients have a direct bearing on the health of a person.

INTERVIEW #1:   An interesting interview with Charlotte Gerson, daughter of Max Gerson, the founder of the Gerson Institute was aired on KCJH radio on January 10, 1995. She told about her father and his method of helping people with different diseases, including cancer, to get well.

She said the following: "Dr Gerson was a physician trained like every other physician, to diagnose and drug their people with medications. He himself was suffering several migraine headaches and none of the drugs were helping him. When he asked his professors and teachers they said, 'Well, this is incurable. You have to live with it.' He said, 'I can't.' So he decided he would have to find his own way how to get well. It was very difficult because there were no directions anywhere until he found in some obscure Italian journal something about a lady with migraine headaches who had benefited from a change of diet."

"He said, 'Now that sounds reasonable. Something I eat is not agreeing with me and is causing pain, nausea, etc. He tried to change his diet and started drinking milk thinking that even a baby can digest milk, but it did not work. So then he felt like fruit and vegetables might be the key. Living in Germany at the time he decided to eat nothing but apples. They were plentiful in all seasons so he ate fresh apples, applesauce, baked apples, apple juice and he got well."

"Based on that information he slowly added one item after another to see what he could handle and what he could not, thus developing what he called his migraine diet. As long as he stayed on it, he had no migraine headaches."

"If patients would come to his office and complain of migraine headaches, he would tell them about his experiment and tell them to try it. They all would come back healed. One day a patient came back to him after four or five weeks and not only were his migraine headaches gone, but also his skin tuberculosis was gone also."

"My father could not believe that. You see he was like a regular physician where one approach only helped one disease. It could not heal two diseases. So he said, 'No, no, it couldn't have been. This is an incurable disease. It must have been something else. But the man showed laboratory proof that indeed he had had skin tuberculosis. And then my father asked if he knew of others with tuberculosis and the man said, 'Yes, at the hospital where I was, there are several.'"

"My father said, 'Send them to me. I will treat them free of charge.' And that is how my father began to help heal tuberculosis. These people recovered. He decided to try and help bone and lung tuberculosis also, and sure enough they recovered. Many of those patients had other problems such as allergies, asthma, kidney disease, migraine, etc., and it turned out that all these problems disappeared also on his program, which consisted of raw food, raw juices, raw salad, steamed vegetables, baked potatoes and such, free of additives, free of chemicals, fats and salt."

"Then he found out that this diet also helped cancer patients. He found out that that animal fats and protein (all animal products), and sodium stimulate tumor growth. Salt is needed for fast cell division for tumor growth, so when you eliminate salt and animal products, and flood the body with essential nutrients and detoxify it, the body starts to heal itself. The immune system is restored, the mineral balances are restored, the liver and all the essential organs start to heal."

Interviewer: "Did the Gerson therapy become very well known because of the tuberculosis, or was it beginning to work with cancer patients, multiple sclerosis, and other degenerative diseases?"

Charlotte: "Well, in Europe the major thing before Dr. Gerson came to America in 1936, it was mainly known because of the tuberculosis work, as well as other things like arthritis and allergies. It was relatively less well-known for cancer because his results at that time were not yet as reliable. He had not yet worked out the importance of leaving off animal proteins. He was still using some, like the yokes of egg, but that was deadly for cancer patients because of the fat content."

Interviewer: "What kind of patients come to you now?"

Charlotte: "Cancer patients who have had some kind of treatment and therapies already. They have gone through radiation and surgeries and unfortunately, in a number of cases, chemo. It is so extremely poisonous and these toxic substances remain in the body and cause trouble. Most of the patients that we receive are terminal with all the treatment they have received, and the cancer is spreading throughout the body. Because of the treatments they have additional damage to deal with. The destruction of the immune system, the damage to the functioning of the organs. We have a real tough situation with almost every single patient, and yet to a large number of patients, fortunately we are still able to achieve healing results. We are not just talking three or six months remission. We are talking five years and up-cured."

"In orthodox medicine sometimes they keep the patient alive, but they are so miserable they wish they were dead, because they are in such terrible condition. It is no quality of life at all. We work for total recovery and most of the time we get it, including such cases of pancreatic cancers, liver, lymphoma. When all the doctors have failed, we have had wonderful results in many cases."

Interviewer: "If somebody comes to your clinic and they have been diagnosed and told they have one month to live with lymphatic cancer, breast cancer or terminally ill with it spreading, they have taken chemotherapy. What do you do with them once they get there?"

Charlotte: "Especially after the chemo, we have to be cautious. Let's assume that they have not had much chemo. We first of all flood the body with nutrients. They get a fresh glass of juice every hour made from organic vegetables: largely carrots, apples, and green salad vegetables. In other words extremely rich in enzymes, minerals, carotenes, vitamins, and all of the things the bodies are so deficient in. If we were to give this in pill form, they are virtually not absorbed or assimilated. You can stuff pills in their mouth, but these nutrients have to go into the cells that are so toxic."

"We also have to detoxify them. The juices help to flush out the poisons and then we also use the caffeine and coffee enemas rectally. Caffeine helps the liver to open up and release from the liver and bile duct the accumulated poisons."

Interviewer: "Can you give us a quick summary of your program for a 14 day period?"

Charlotte: "Fresh juice every hour, which includes one ounce of orange juice, 4 of those juices are made with various greens with a little apple juice, and the rest are carrot and apple, and of course, we serve carrot juice alone also. All fruits and vegetables are organic. Then the patient receives three full vegetarian meals on top of the juices. Then they receive extensive vitamin, enzyme, and mineral supplements, a boost of liver extract, B12 and liver capsules. (Of course, you know, the liver is the key organ in the body responsible for healing)."

INTERVIEW #2: The next interview was in May of 1995, with Dr. Lorraine Day, who is an internationally acclaimed orthopedic trauma surgeon, best-selling author for 15 years, on the faculty of the University of California of San Francisco School of Medicine as an Associate Professor, and Vice Chairman of the Department of Orthopedics. She had breast cancer and made some radical choices, which she will talk about in this interview. She makes some rather startling statements and introduces her remarks by the following information:

Dr. Day: "Everything I say about breast cancer applied to all cancers. Cancers are not different one from another even though we in orthodox medicine have always told patients we have to know not only exactly the kind of cancers you have, but exactly the category within that kind of cancer because then we can treat it, and target these special kinds of agents that actually destroy your immune system. All cancer is a disease of the immune system, whether it shows up in your colon or in your breast or in your prostate, it is all the same. Cancer does not hit you like lightning out of the sky. We really in most part do it to ourselves, but the other thing is that the same blood that circulates through the tumor circulates through the rest of the body."

Interviewer: "What did you do when you found out you had the breast cancer?"

Dr. Day: "First of all I should tell the people that I had a biopsy and had the lump removed to make sure that it was cancer. The doctor who removed it said, 'We could not get it all without taking off your breast.' I had refused to have my breast removed, so I said, 'Leave those cancer cells in.' All of us have cancer cells in our body everyday, but if our immune system is working properly, it destroys those cancer cells. I knew what I needed to do was to feed my immune system and nourish it. And what I did was a basic three point plan."

"*Number I*: I decided to get good highly nutritious food into my body in the form of vegetable juices, and organically grown foods without pesticides."

"*Number two*: I had to get the toxins out of my body. America is dying in their own toxins. We are all constipated because we are eating too much sugar, too much highly processed food, and too much fat. So everything sits around in the intestines for days and days and it putrefies, and puts off toxins which we re-absorb into our bodies. So we have to have a fast transit time from the time we eat until we get rid of the waste material. And the way I started doing that was not only using colon cleansers, but enemas. I started off with five enemas a day. Colonic enemas are also an excellent way to clean out the colon of all the debris that has been in there for years and years, which is stuck to the inside of the colon."

"*Number three*: I tried to get the known toxins out of my local environment. Look under the kitchen sink, bathroom sink for all those chemicals that are putting off fumes we are breathing in."

"I also added essiac tea, aloe vera, laetrile, powdered barley green, and wheat grass."

Interviewer: "What are the draw backs of radiation and chemotherapy?"

Dr. Day: "I have been a very conventional physician all of my life. I have never been on the fringe of medicine. I have been in the heart of academic medicine and served on the faculty of the University of California. We have been brainwashed for years that there are only three ways to treat cancer. In fact there is booklet put out by the state of California for the AMA signed by Governor Pete Wilson, which says there are only three ways to treat cancer: chemotherapy, radiation, or surgery, (which is mainly mutilating surgery-cut it out). I'm a surgeon, but we as surgeons are really good about these things. What we say is, 'Well, if your tonsils bother you, let's cut them out. If your appendices bothers you, let's cut them out. If your prostate bothers you, cut it off, if your breast is not working right, cut it off. What do you do if you get a headache? What we need to do is made the organs work properly. So I said, 'Well, now, let's see. We as physicians have been telling people for years that radiation is bad for you because it can cause cancer. We say, 'Don't get too many x-rays,' and yet they tell women, 'We've got to give you x-rays to see if you have cancer with the mammogram, and if you do have cancer we have got to give you huge doses of what we told you to avoid because it causes cancer.'"

"Now that doesn't make any sense to me. I know chemo therapy are poisons. In fact the first director of chemo therapy in the United States was the doctor who was in charge of chemical warfare in World War II. Those same warfare agents that are meant to kill people, like nitrogen mustard, was one of the first therapy agents. The developers of chemo therapy said, 'Well, these kill people, so why don't we give them to cancer patients and maybe we can just kill part of them.'"

"The fact is, it generally kills all of them. What it does do is kill a lot of cancer cells, but it kills so many good cells and it kills so much of the immune system that when the cancer comes back, which it almost always does, because you never kill all the cells, the immune system is so destroyed that it cannot kill those remaining cancer cells and the cancer consumes you. That is why people seem like they go into remission for a year and then it comes back and they die. Radiation and chemotherapy both kill cells. Radiation burns. It kills cells. It kills indiscriminately. No matter what your doctor will tell you about how targeted it is, it kills cells indiscriminately. That is why your hair falls out when you have chemotherapy. I have never known anybody who had cancer of the hair follicles, but yet your hair falls out."

"The body is a wonderful organism. God made it to heal itself. If we just stand back and don't destroy it, it will heal itself if we treat it properly. Now, your doctor does not know what I'm telling you. I did not know this 10 years ago. If I'd have gotten breast cancer 10 years ago, I would have gone the conventional medicine route because I believed it, because we have been so totally brainwashed, and this information about alternative therapies is kept out of the medical libraries. It is not readily available there, but you can find certain articles if you search for it. In fact, after I found out about alternative medicines, I went through the medical literature and I was able to confirm that many herbs and various other things do decrease tumor size. It is all in there, but they never bring it out to you, and they encourage conventional doctors to ridicule this as quackery because how could anything you eat be related to your health?"

INTERVIEW #3: The next interview aired on KCJH radio station during the program *Heathline*, was with Dr. Contreras on April 4, 1995. He is the head of the Contreras Hospital in Mexico, where they have treated over 40,000 patients.

Interviewer: "Give us an introduction about the work at your hospital."

Dr. Contreras: "My father began this work about 31 years ago. He was working very diligently treating cancer patients in an orthodox manner, and he felt there needed to be a change. The Lord showed him that the doctors were not taking into account the emotional and spiritual needs of the patient. While he was visiting Ephesus and saw the ruins of a sanitarium or hospital, the guide told him (because he knew that my dad was a prominent doctor from Mexico), that the way it worked 1000 years before Christ is that the patient would come in and be evaluated emotionally, spiritually, and physically. Originally medicine was geared to be that way, but since then we have become very scientific and technologically oriented we have forgotten about those needs. He felt that was the main reason why we were failing so terribly, especially with cancer patients, or any patient with chronic illnesses. He came back to begin his work in trying to see the needs of his patients physically, spiritually, and emotionally. He really saw the need to try to gain the patient for Christ. He felt like eternal life was even more important than physical needs. He put it to himself as a mission more than a medical service. We have seen a lot of miracles that have come more than through medical ministrations really through spiritual ministrations, because lastly we have to accept even if we have a lot of experience about medicine we have to accept the only one that cures is God. We have been blessed not only to minister to our patients healing methods, but also the Word of God."

Interviewer: "How does your clinic differ from a hospital in America? What approach do you take?"

Dr. Contreras: "We look into alternate medicine because statistics show that more people die because of the treatment against cancer than cancer itself. We choose the best of either alternative, orthodox, or no therapy, and individualize treatment for each patient."

Interviewer: "Tell us about the son of Max Factor, one of your patients who received help."

Dr. Contreras: "He was 47 years old when he came to us about eight years ago from England, after being treated with chemo therapy for a very advanced cancer of the colon with matasitis to the liver and lungs. They told him there was nothing more that could be done, so he and his family traveled by plane here in a very devastating condition, almost in a coma condition."

"My father decided the best thing for him was prayer and fasting. So a number of us started to pray and fast. We also started with a treatment, giving it directly to his liver, because the liver was the one that was so damaged. Thank God he is alive now, completely cured, and it has been five years without any tumor activity."

Dr. Gersen and Dr. Cotreras both agree that a healthy liver is essential for good health. Dr. Michael Murray, who is an author and a naturepathic doctor, said the following during his live interview on *Healthline*, May 16, 1995. He said, "The liver is the major organ in metabolism. It controls fatty metabolism, protein metabolism, and carbohydrate metabolism. When it is not working up to par, when it is being over-loaded, (because it is also responsible for detoxifying body hormones as well as environmental pollutants), it just doesn't work as properly and people can suffer from low-energy level depression, a general malay, or they may not be able to properly assimilate the food that they eat, so it really causes a lot of problems. People can help by drinking enough water, by making sure they do not over consume sugar or saturated fat. We should eat a diet that is very rich in plant foods because plant foods are very rich in anti-oxidant, which helps the liver function better and also the source of fiber which promotes good bile flow. The liver determines a person's level of health. If it is not working properly it is impossible to have good energy and health."

He suggests taking the supplement, *Liv-a-tox* with your daily food. It is an enzymatic therapy which contains nutrients that are essential for proper liver function. These nutrients are utilized by the liver in its detoxification reactions.

The National Cancer Institute gave a list of things to do to prevent cancer in the *McCall's* magazine, November 1984 issue. A recent survey by the NCI shows that 46 percent of all Americans incorrectly believe that there is nothing they can do to prevent cancer. You can help yourself. The NCI suggests you take the following steps:

1.   Avoid too much sunlight, particularly if you are fair-skinned. This precaution could prevent more than 90 percent of cases of the commonest form of cancer: nonmelanoma skin cancer.

2.   Don't smoke. Smoking causes cancer, and it also can increase the risk you incur from other carcinogens in the environment.

3.   Change your diet. The NCI has released dietary guidelines they say will reduce your risk of getting certain kinds of cancer. Eat foods low in fat and low enough in calories to keep you trim. Eat more fresh fruits and vegetables high in vitamins A and C and fiber, such as spinach, sweet potatoes, cabbage, broccoli, tomatoes, cauliflower, carrots, peaches, strawberries, cantaloupe, grapefruit, honeydew melons, potatoes, beans, peas and seeds. Also include whole-grain breads and cereals in your daily diet. Choose lead red meats, fish and poultry.

4.   (NCI says drink only one or two alcoholic beverages a day.   I, the author, say don't drink any) . . . Excessive drinking has been linked to mouth, throat, esophagus and liver cancers.

5.   Don't ask for an X-ray if your doctor or dentist doesn't recommend it. If you need an X-ray, ask for X-ray shields to protect other parts of your body.

6.   Avoid excessive exposure to chemicals of any kind.

7.   If you are a woman in menopause, discuss estrogen use and dosage with your doctor,

and use it only as long as needed. High-dose estrogen has been linked to an increase in cancer of the lining of the womb among women who take it for menopausal systoms.

I received the following testimony from Kaye Singleton, one of my friends, who chose a different route than chemotherapy and radiation. She says the following:

"January 17, 1995, I was diagnosed with breast cancer, and on January 30, 1995, I had a mastectomy on the right breast. Oncologist suggested that even though there was no further evidence of cancer in my body that I take chemotherapy, radiation, and tamoxathin as a preventive for reoccurrence of cancer in the next five years. After praying about this decision, reading, and counseling with a minister and his wife, I felt that God was leading me in another direction. My minister friends took me to a health food store where the owner had over 100 tumors in his lungs 12 years prior, and had recovered and watched them all disappear on x-rays by following the Macrobiotic Diet.

"Macrobiotic in Japanese simply means "long life." The Japanese have what they call "Yin" and "Yang." If you eat too many "Yang foods you will be too tight. On the other hand if you eat too many "Yin" foods you will be too lose. They believe in eating balanced and not swinging to either side. It consists of seven primary food groups as follows:

WHOLE GRAIN CEREAL: Rice, wheat, barley, oats, millet, corn, buckwheat, or rye grains are the principle food in the macrobiotic diet. Grains should be consumed at every meal and comprise from 40-60% of the total volume of food eaten every day.

VEGETABLE: The total daily food volume of vegetables should be 20-40% Vegetables should be as fresh as you can obtain.

SOUPS: Approximately 5% of the total volume is suggested. Soup stocks are made with either miso, a fermented soybean puree, or tamari soy sauce.

BEANS: The daily volume should be 10%, depending on your personal protein requirement.

SEA VEGETABLES: These are an important ingredient in macrobiotic cooking. It takes some getting used to, but are an important source of trace minerals. They are used mostly in cooking beans and soup stock, but are also used in vegetable dishes.

ANIMAL PROTEIN: Fish in the recommended source. The varieties of fish used in preference are white meat varieties and those with a low fat content. Red meat and chicken is prohibited, because of the chemicals used for processing.

SUPPLEMENTAL FOODS: This group includes fruits and nuts.

BEVERAGES: Spring water, non-stimulant teas, fruit or vegetable juices (no sugar or salt added), and if you like coffee, Roma is a grain coffee that is good." (So says, Kaye Singleton, who has no cancer cells in her body, March 20, 1996.)

Chapter 11

Keep Slim and Trim

Why would a person want to have an ideal weight and remain at said weight? There are several reasons.

Number one: it is a proven fact that people feel better when they are not overweight. It helps them not to feel so sluggish and they can mobilize better.

Number two: There is a psychological reason involved. People who look good and feel good about themselves physically are more prone to be confident people. They are not always worrying about how they look, so they are able to focus their attention on other people and their needs. They can become involved in many interesting projects, be able to travel easier, go and do, instead of hiding behind closed doors, becoming introverted, and satisfied only by food consumption.

Number three: People are more apt to harbor disease when they are overweight. Heart trouble and other diseases many times can be helped by losing extra weight among other things. Karen A. Wilson related to readers of the *Good Housekeeping*, March 1996 issue, "Why Big *Isn't* Beautiful." She told how she reached the weight of 330 pounds comforted by the message that big was beautiful until one day when she went to the bathroom, looked down, and saw the toilet filled with blood. She was terrified. When she finally went to the doctor, they found she had precancerous cells in the lining of her uterus. After surgery, she learned that the cancer had spread to the uterine muscles and lymph channels in the pelvic area.

When she first got the diagnosis, her doctor had told her about the link between obesity and endometrial cancer. She said during the weeks of radiation treatment that followed, she read everything she could get her hands on about the subject. She learned that "fat cells produce their own estrogen and in seriously overweight women, all this extra estrogen can run amok, causing the uterine lining to overgrow and possibly become cancerous."

The first thing that a person must do is to have a physical check-up and make sure that it is not an imbalance that is causing them to gain weight. After that is ruled out, there should be a choosing of an ideal weight according to height, bone structure and other important details. There are many kinds of diets on the bookstands that promise miracles, but to lose weight, you must have will-power to stick with the adopted lifestyle. At the end of this chapter is crash a diet given to my husband quite a few years ago, that originated from the Mayo Clinic and is reputed to guarantee a quick weight loss from 6-10 pounds in 4 days.

Whatever way you decide to loose weight and get down to your ideal weight is your choice entirely, but making the choice and sticking with it is what is important. After you lose your weight, the problem many times becomes maintaining it.

There are several ways to stay at an ideal weight. One way, of course, is being aware of what is eaten and practicing moderation. Example: instead of eating 2 pieces of strawberry pie try eating slower, savoring each bite and eat only one. It is being aware that one can eat a good portion of vegetables, salads, fish and chicken without gaining weight, if they are prepared properly.

More than being temperate or eating in moderation, I have discovered a secret, which would help people, so that they would not have to fight the battle of the bulge as much. It is simply called the 12-hour fast. "Ugh!" you say, who wants to fast. Although fasting is recommended by some physicians, the 12 hour fast I am talking about is very simply done and you still eat three meals a day. Let me explain, If you have your last meal in the evening at 7:00 p.m., then your next meal would be at 7:00

a.m. the next morning or later. In other words you fast 12 hours each night. If your last meal is at 12:00 midnight, then your next meal would be 12:00 noon. Remember, later eating contributes to settled fat because there is no exercising. The late meals most always go to fat. If you have to have something, eat light. Fish would be better than Prime Rib or a salad would be better than a hamburger with fries.

Some people become so stuffed with food they become bloated on needless calories, they overwork their digestive system, thereby contributing to health problems. The fact of digestion is taken into consideration in the recommendation of the 12 hour fast.

Digestion is the process by which food is broken down into smaller particles, or molecules, for use in the human body. This breakdown makes it possible for the smaller digested particles to pass through the intestinal wall into the blood stream. Digestion begins in the mouth. Chewing is very important to good digestion, for two reasons: when chewed food is ground into fine particles, the digestive juices, which contain enzymes, can react more easily. As the food is chewed, it is moistened and mixed with saliva which contains the enzyme ptyalin. Ptyalin changes some of the starches to sugar. After the food is swallowed, it passes through the esophagus into the stomach. In the stomach it is thoroughly mixed with more digestive juices by a vigorous chewy motion. This churning motion is caused by the contraction of strong muscles in the walls if the stomach. The digestive juice in the stomach is called gastric juice. It contains hydrochloric acid and the enzyme pepsin. The gastric juice begins the digestion of protein foods such as meat, eggs and milk. Starches and sugars in fats are not digested by the gastric juice. The food remains in the stomach for 2-5 hours, depending on the types of food. Food which has been churned, partly digested, and changed to a thick liquid in the stomach is called chyme. Chyme passes from the stomach into the small intestine.

In the small intestine, the digestive process is completed on the partly digested food by pancreatic juice, intestinal juice, and bile. The pancreatic juice is produced by the pancreas and pours into the small intestine through a tube or duct. The intestinal juice is produced by the walls of the small intestine. Bile is produced in the liver, stored in the gall bladder, and flows into the small intestine through the bile duct. It helps the body digest and absorb fat.

When the food is completely digested, it is absorbed by tiny blood lymph vessels in the walls of the small intestine. It is then carried into the circulation for nourishment of the body. Food particles are small enough to pass through the walls of the intestine and blood vessels only when they are completely digested .

Almost no digestion takes place in the large intestine. It stores waste food product and absorbs small amounts of water and minerals. The waste materials that accumulate in the large intestine are roughage that cannot be digested in the body. This is eliminated from the body from time to time. What is interesting is that after a regular meal is eaten, the last part of that meal finally leaves the body 48 hours later in normal digestion.

An example of the digestive cycle taken from *The World Encyclopedia* is as follows:

First day	6:00 p.m.	Dinner is eaten
	6:01	First food enters stomach
	10:30 p.m.	stomach is empty
	1:00 a.m.	Food has passed through small intestine
Second day	6:00 p.m.	First waste ready to leave large intestine
Third day	6:00 p.m.	48 hours after meal, last waste ready to leave large intestine

Note: This is eating a normal diet. If a person is eating only fruit, then the digestion system is speeded up, and this schedule would change.

It stands to reason that if a person keeps stuffing themselves with food, before the body can properly digest the previous food, there will be much excess. The body needs a 12 hour rest for health reasons also. The colon that becomes clogged from overeating and improper digestion will cause other diseases because of the toxic waste that is lying dormant in it.

By adhering to the 12 hour principle you not only are keeping your weight down but you are prolonging your life. The heart then does not have to overwork trying to digest an overload of food that was consumed an hour before retiring.

Four Day Crash Diet (from the Mayo Clinic)
Author's modification: If you are not eating meat, you could substitute a tofu burger or meat substitute in place of the steak.

Breakfast for each day is the same: 1/2 grapefruit, or 4 oz. grapefruit juice and black coffee. (I would forego the coffee).

First Day:
    Lunch
    4 oz. broiled steak (trimmed of all fat) *or meat substitute.*
    Lettuce & tomato salad
    Apple

    Dinner
    2 Hard boiled eggs
    String beans
    1/2 grapefruit or 4 oz. grapefruit juice

Second Day: *Lunch*
1 broiled lamb chop
Plain lettuce salad
4 oz. tomato juice

Dinner
Squash, cauliflower, string beans
Apple sauce

Third Day: *Lunch*
4 oz. broiled steak *or meat substitute*
Lettuce Salad
Apple

Dinner
Chicken broiled without skin
Stewed tomatoes
4 oz. prune juice

Fourth Day: *Lunch*
2 scrambled eggs
String beans
Tomato juice

Dinner
4 oz. broiled steak *or meat substitute*
Lettuce Salad
Pineapple

Note: All servings are 4 oz. No dressing on salad. Use seasoned salt or lemon juice.

Judith Rodin, Ph.D., wrote an article entitled, *Taming the Hunger Hormone.* She asked the question, "Is insulin the key to weight control?" She writes, "Insulin is the body's fuel regulator. It guides sugar and fat from the blood stream into the body's cells. Muscle cells use the fuel for energy; fat cells store it. Diabetics suffer because they don't have enough insulin, and their blood sugar builds up.

"But recent studies have brought some startling news: Insulin affects the brain as profoundly as the body. The same hormone that dispatches your food tells you to eat. High insulin levels make you hungry, make you eat more and make sweets taste better. Insulin, in fact, appears to have much more to do with appetite than your level of blood sugar does. When you gain weight, your body's cells become less sensitive to insulin, and you compensate by producing more of the hormone. This extra insulin can build fat tissue, and it can keep you hungry." After testing 20 normal-weight men and women who had insulin and glucose added to their blood every half-hour, they came up with these results: "When we pumped our subjects with insulin, they became hungrier and liked sweet tastes more. And when we gave them a liquid-formula lunch at the end of the experiment, they drank more than people whose insulin had been kept moderately low. Changing levels of blood sugar, on the other hand, had no effect on their appetite or craving for sweets"

They then asked another question and experimented further, "Do some foods boost insulin levels higher than others? And do they make people eat more? The answer is yes to both."

Rodin writes, "My colleagues and I decided to check out the folklore that sweets trigger eating binges, and to see if insulin could be the cause. Psychologist Lynn Spitzer compared two types of sugar, fructose (found in fruits) and glucose (used in many prepared foods and baked goods). These two have the same number of calories, the same taste and the same chemical formula, but a slight difference in molecular structure gives them very different effects on the body."

Dr. Rodin continues, "When you eat glucose, your blood sugar rises sharply, and your body produces more insulin to get glucose from your blood to your cells. Your blood glucose then drops quickly, but your insulin level stays higher for two or three hours. Fructose produces a much slower, and more moderate, rise in both blood sugar and insulin. (Table sugar is a mix of glucose and fructose, but for some reason its effects are like those of pure glucose.)

"It seemed to us that people should be famished two hours after a shot of glucose, when their insulin would still be high and their blood sugar low. But we thought that fructose would tame their appetite for hours at a time. An experiment proved us right."

This experiment proves that a candy bar will make you more hungry an hour later, than if you would have eaten an apple. The fruit would help tame the appetite; whereas, the candy would increase the appetite.

American Health published a "glyceic index" of foods, developed by Dr. David Jenkins at the University of Toronto. This list shows how quickly different foods boost blood sugar and raise your insulin. Foods with a high number act the most like glucose, leading to an insulin jump. Foods with a low index give a slow rise in blood sugar, fructose, fruits, complex carbohydrates.

Sugars

Fructose	20
Glucose	100

Pasta, Rice

Whole-wheat spaghetti	42
White spaghetti	50
Brown Rice	66
White Rice	72

Cereals

Oatmeal	49
Shredded Wheat	67
Cornflakes	80

Fruits

Apples	39
Oranges	40
Bananas	62
Raisins	64

Root Vegetables

Sweet Potatoes	48
White Potatoes	70
Carrots	92
Parsnips	97

Dairy Products

Skim Milk	32
Ice Cream	36
Yogurt	36

Peas and Beans

Soybeans	15
Lentils	29
Kidney Beans	29

Miscellaneous

Peanuts	13
Potato chips	51
Pastry	59
Mars Bar	68

It is apparent from the above chart which foods are best for the health of the body.

Chapter 12

Cleansing the Body

Fasting is as old as the early civilization, but is often misunderstood, misused and neglected. Fasting is not starving and it does not exhaust the body's reserves. There is quite a difference between starving and fasting. One of the best ways to fast is to consume only water, no food. In fact, water is a faster's best friend. Fasting is a great way to rid the body of poisonous toxins. The kidneys are a miracle working machine. Outside of the brain, the kidneys are perhaps the most complex organ of the body.

When you go on a fast, you allow the digestive systems in your body to rest. Thus the cleansing capacity of the lungs, liver, kidneys, and the skin is intensified. The accumulated toxins in your body from food additives and wrong eating, when in a fast, are released into the blood stream and then expelled.

167

Water is a great flushing agent in fasting. it gets rid of the toxins and waste material that build up when fatty tissue is "burned".

Another sign of toxic elimination is that you will notice a coating on your tongue. Fasting gives your digestive organs a rest so that its energies can be devoted to cleansing your body of impurities. As these wastes are eliminated during your fast, you will find you have increased energy, keener alertness, and a brighter disposition towards life. Fasting does many good things for you. Here are some of the benefits of fasting.

- Helps you sleep better
- Gives the digestive system a rest
- Regulates bowels
- Makes you more alert
- Lowers your blood pressure
- Helps heal the body
- Slows aging process
- Helps you feel better
- Helps you gain control over weight
- Helps sharpen the brain and mental processes
- Helps you see things in better perspective
- Creates a greater kinship with God and spiritual things

I have already recommended the 12 hour nightly fast, but it would be healthy physically and spiritually for you to fast one day a week. If you want to eat every day that is possible and still fast a 24 hour day during the week.

Example: The last meal on Tuesday would be 6:00 for the evening meal, and the next meal would be 6:00 Wednesday evening.

Some people have said that it takes an amount of time equal to the fasting time to recuperate from the effects of fasting. That is, one month of fasting will require one month of recuperating. I disagree. If a fast is undertaken properly, one should feel better, stronger, and healthier than when the fast began.

Juice Fasting

Dr. Paavo Airola tells a story in his book, *Juice Fasting,* that is worth retelling. A 54 year old woman went to his Spa in a desperate condition. For years she had worked in the field of health and beauty and had operated a figure control salon in Los Angeles and helped countless men and women to better health. When she reached age 45 her health and her looks started to deteriorate. She began putting on weight and, in spite of her rigid program of exercises, was not able to control it.

Signs of premature aging appeared suddenly. Her hair started to turn gray, wrinkles appeared on her face, and in addition she felt stiffness and pain in her fingers, elbows and shoulders, which was diagnosed by her doctor as early symptoms of rheumatoid arthritis. Also, her complexion began to deteriorate rapidly. Her skin was dry and lifeless, and patches of psoriasis appeared behind her ears. She felt exhausted most of the time and lost interest in her work. She had developed an uncontrollable appetite and was putting on pounds each week. She sold her business and tried to get a job as a health, beauty, and personality counselor in a home for young girls, but was turned down because of her overweight.

This incident was a great shock to her and a turning point in her life. She had noticed that some of her friends started to avoid her and some even felt sorry for her. Her personality had changed. She had grown critical of everyone and everything, and her temper was getting worse and worse.

Dr. Airola says that many women are in similar situations, and some of them blame their *condition* on *the change of life*, but this woman decided to do something about it. Although she had worked most of her life in a figure control and beauty field, she never thought much about nutrition and what role it plays in health. When she entered Dr. Airola's Spa, she was 54, weighed 184 pounds, and looked like 60. He outlined a three month program for her. First, one month of fasting on juices. Then a controlled raw food diet with special vitamins and mineral supplements for four weeks. After that, two more weeks of fasting and two weeks of dieting.

She followed the program religiously. She received two glasses of diluted fruit juice, two glasses of vegetable juice, one glass of vegetable broth, and 2 cups of herb tea each day. In addition, she drank one glass of mineral water and any amount of plain water she wanted. She took long walks, up to 5 miles a day, and was advised to take enemas twice a day, morning and evening.

At the end of the first month, she had lost 28 pounds. She lost an additional 12 pounds during the 30 days of raw food diet. She ate 3 meals of the most delicious raw vegetables and tropical fruits each day in addition to the regular juices. She also took lecithin, kelp, brewer's yeast and vitamins B, C, A, and E. By the end of the three months, she had a total weight loss of 52 pounds.

When she left the spa, she weighed 132 pounds, and had gone from size 20 to size 12. Her arthritis and psoriasis had disappeared, and instead of feeling old, tired, apathetic, discouraged and disillusioned, she now was filled with energy and enthusiasm, full of exciting plans for the future. Her vitality and enthusiasm were limitless and the change in her appearance was miraculous.

She was amazed that her collagen was strengthened and the elasticity in her skin was restored; her new-cell building and cell repair accelerated, and muscle tone improved, even though she had lost so much weight in such a short time. Her skin was tighter than before, her wrinkles were less noticeable and her previously muddy and gray complexion had acquired a fresh radiant look.

Juice fasting is one of the most effective ways to restore your health and rejuvenate your body. The aging begins when your normal process of cell regeneration and rebuilding slows down. This slowdown can be caused by the accumulation of waste products in the tissues which interferes with the nourishment of the cells.

How can the mere abstinence from food solids accomplish such remarkable results? During a prolonged fast (after the first three days), your body will live on its own substance. Your body will first decompose and burn those cells and tissues which are diseased, damaged, aged or dead. "In fasting, your body feeds itself on the most impure and inferior materials, such as dead cells and morbid accumulations, tumors, abscesses, damaged tissues, fat deposits, etc. Dr. Buchingr Sr., one of the greatest fasting authorities in the world, calls fasting, a 'refuse disposal,' a 'burning of rubbish.' These dead cells and inferior tissues are consumed and utilized first. The essential tissues and vital organs, the glands, the nervous systems and the brain are spared." [1]

"During fasting, while the old cells and diseased tissues are decomposed and burned, the building of new, healthy cells is stimulated and speeded up. This may seem unbelievable, since no nourishment or only a limited amount of nourishment (during a juice fast) is supplied . . . During a juice fast, the eliminative and cleansing capacity of the eliminative organs-lungs, liver, kidneys, bowels and skin-is greatly increased, and masses of accumulated metabolic wastes and toxins are quickly expelled...The nervous system is rejuvenated; mental powers are improved; glandular chemistry and hormonal secretions are stimulated; biochemical and mineral balance in the tissues is normalized." [2]

Dr. Airola gives the following four scientific justifications of juice fasting:

1. Raw juices, as well as freshly made vegetable broths, are rich in vitamins, minerals, trace elements and enzymes.

2. These vital elements are very easily assimilated directly into the bloodstream, without putting a strain on the digestive system; thus they do not disrupt the healing and rejuvenating process of autolysis, or self-digestion.

3. The nutritive elements from the juices are extremely beneficial in normalizing all the body processes, supplying needed elements for the body's own healing activity and cell regeneration, and, thus, speeding the recovery.

4. Generous amounts of minerals in the juices, particularly in the vegetable broth, help to restore the biochemical and mineral balance in the tissues and cells. Mineral imbalance in the tissues is one of the main causes of diminished oxygenation, which leads to disease and the premature aging of cells.

Chapter 13

Brain Power

The brain, as already stated, is capable of storing as much as ten times more information than there is in the library of Congress, with its 17 million volumes.

The B vitamins, especially cholene and B6, play an important role in maintaining memory. The amino acids are also very important. A diet that is nutritionally deficient and high in processed foods, junk foods, and fried foods may cause poor memory and concentration. A hormone imbalance and certain glandular disorders may also cause memory loss.

The Artesian Health Store in Stockton, California, gave me the chart on the following page, which can be helpful for those interested in increasing their memory. They have divided it into three categories: Very important, Important, and Helpful.

Nutrients

Very Important		
Supplement	**Suggested Dosage**	**Comments**
Choline	100 mg 3 times daily	Increases amount of aceltylcholine, the message carrier of the brain.
Niacin and niacinamide (B3)	As directed on label	Aids in function of the brain and blood flow.
Vitamin B complex	100 mg daily	
B6 (pyridoxine	50 mg 3 times daily	For improved memory
Pantothenic Acid (B5)	50 mg 3 times daily	Helps transformation of choline to acetylcholine.
Vitamin C	3,000 to 10,000 mg	Powerful antioxidant. Improves circulation.

Important		
Supplement	**Suggested Dosage**	**Comments**
L-Glutamine & L-phenylalanine & aspartic acid (amino acids)	As directed on label	Necessary for normal **brain function**
Lecithin	1 Tbsp with meals or 2 capsules with meals	Improves brain function high in choline and inosital)

176

Helpful		
Supplement	**Suggested Dosage**	**Comments**
Coenzyme Q10	100 mg daily	Improvesbrain oxygenation
DMG (Gluconic from DaVinci Labs)	As directed on label	Improvesbrain oxygenation
Gerovital H-3 (GH-3) or Aslavital	As directed on label	From Romania-good for the elderly.
RNA-DNA	As directed on label	Increases energy production for memory transfer in the brain. Caution: Do not use if you have elevated serum uric acid or gout.

Herbs that are considered helpful for the brain are anise, blue cohosh, ginkgo biloba extract, ginseng, rosemary, and also bee pollen. The following foods should be consumed often: whole grains, tofu, farm eggs, legumes, wheat germ, soybeans, fish, brewer's yeast, nuts, millet, brown rice, and raw foods. Do not consume refined sugar (these "turn off" the brain).

An all-carbohydrate meal will adversely affect the memory. For a better memory, combine complex carbohydrates with foods comprised of 10 percent protein and 10 percent essential fats.

Ginkgo biloba: The Artesian Health Store of Stockton, California, gave me an article written by Dr. Michael Murray, who is a practicing physician in Kirkland, Washington, and is regarded as a leading medical researcher in the naturopathic profession. It is entitled "Nutritional Information on Ginkgo Biloba Extract." He writes the following: "A remarkable tree is the source of great hope for aging patients with signs and symptoms of insufficient blood supply to the brain. These symptoms include senility, short-term memory loss, vertigo, headache, ringing in the ears, lack of vigilance and depression. These symptoms of decreased cerebral blood flow are extremely common in the geriatric population due to the presence of atherosclerotic cardiovascular disease.

"The Ginkgo is the world's oldest living tree. Ginkgo's pharmacological activity is due to its high content of terpenes, flavonoids, pro-anthocyanidins and Ginkgo Heterosides (flavoglycosides). A Ginkgo Bilboba extract (G.B.E.) has demonstrated remarkable pharmacological action on different parts of the circulatory and nervous system (arteries, capillaries, veins and heart). Its actions include enhancing energy production, increasing cellular glucose intake and inhibiting platelet aggregation.

"Ginkgo Biloba Extract also promotes radical scavenging activity, increased blood flow to the brain, and improved transmission of nerve signals . . . Furthermore, since G.B.E. improves some aspects of neural transmission, it may be effective in some cases of senility including the early states of Alzheimer's Disease.

"The standard dose is 40 mg three times daily. (so writes Dr. Michael Murray)."

Although the adult brain is only about two percent of body weight, it demands 15 percent of cardiac output and 20-30 percent of resting metabolic rate. Most of the energy expended is used by ongoing chemical processes that produce the brain's electrical energy. The brain depends on a continuous supply of oxygen and glucose fuel.

The brain uses 25 percent of the body's total oxygen intake. This is carried to it in the blood at a rate of 1 1/2 pints per minute. Ten seconds without this supply results in unconsciousness and five minutes more can turn someone into a vegetable. One hundred ten grams of glucose (blood sugar) are required each day at a constant level of 70-100 milligrams per deciliter of blood. Hypoglycemia, low blood sugar, results as glucose levels dip below 70 mg-deciliter, while coma and possible brain damage is the result when levels drop to 8 mg/100 ml of blood.

Besides oxygen and glucose from carbohydrate, the brain uses protein, fat, water and nearly all the vitamins and minerals. Certain nerve cells are insulated with myelin. This is made up of cholesterol and fatty acids. Neutrons enclosed by myelin are capable of transmitting impulses as fast as 270 mph.

The fatty acids are polyunsaturated. Research conducted at the university of Toronto indicates that this kind of fat which is better for our hearts is also better for memory and learning.

As stated on the chart, *choline*, is one of the best nutrients for the brain. Choline cannot be made in the brain but must be synthesized by the liver or supplied in the diet. Acetylcholine is then metabolized by the brain based on a system of supply and demand. Eggs, fish, liver, nutritional yeast (brewer's yeast), beans (especially soybeans), nuts and grains provide major food sources of choline in the form of lecithin. It would be difficult to obtain sufficient amounts of choline for therapeutic measures from food sources.

Lecithin is found in all living cells. It has been a popular health food supplement since Adelle Davis recommended it in her book, *Let's Get Well,* for the treatment of heart disease, diabetes, multiple sclerosis, psoriasis, nephritis and weight reduction back in 1965. In supplement form it is commonly used to improve conditions involving high cholesterol and atherosclerosis, heart disease, gallstones, liver cirrhosis and blood clotting disorders. In the body it is necessary for proper fat utilization, nerve health, memory and learning.

The presence of the B-complex vitamins, vitamins A and C as well as certain mineral elements is absolutely vital to proper brain function. Because the type of unsaturated fat found in the brain is highly susceptible to oxidation, this indicates a need for antioxidant nutrients including vitamin E and selenium. Iron, zinc, iodine, chromium, molybdenum and boron along with copper and manganese have all been mentioned as important to brain function. This is why it is important to eat a well-balanced diet of fresh, unprocessed foods and take a daily multi-vitamin/mineral supplement.

Not only is it important to eat well and take proper supplements, but it is important to exercise. Exercise brings additional oxygen to the brain and is a good way to deal with stress (stress is reported to be one of the most severe deterrents to proper brain function). Writing for *Muscle & Fitness*, Jerry Brainum calls exercise the "stress antidote" and lists the chief benefits of exercise to brain function:

1. Exercise neutralizes many of the excessive by-products of stress reactions.

2. Exercise stimulates the secretion of natural tranquilizers in the brain (endorphins).

3. Exercise potentiates the production of neurotransmitters.

Challenging your brain is another way to improve brain function. Research indicates that brain stimulation promotes new projections from the existing nerve cells. You can stimulate your brain by any activity that requires deep concentration such as reading and memory games.

Chapter 14

A Healthy Heart

Throughout the book, there are many health tips for the heart. Although diet is considered the first line of treatment and one of the very important changes people can make both to alleviate and to prevent heart problems, there are a number of nutrients available in supplement form which enhance heart health and reduce cholesterol levels. Siri Khalsa, health counselor, states in *Nutrition News,* "Elevated serum cholesterol is the most consistent and frequently occurring of all the risk factors. Studies show that as cholesterol declines, the risk of heart attack and stroke drops significantly. For every one percent reduction in blood cholesterol, heart attack risk decreases by two percent."

Niacin is the most effective of the cholesterol lowering supplements. It raises HDL cholesterol while lowering both LDL cholesterol and triglycerides. Lipid research expert, Scott Grundy,

M.D., published a report in 1981, of an experiment which he conducted with twelve participants, all considered at risk for heart attack. They each took one gram of niacin three times daily for one month. At the end of that short period of time, their cholesterol levels had dropped an average of 22 percent and their triglycerides, 52 percent. According to Cara East, Grundy's colleague at the University of Texas Health Science Center, niacin in megadoses works by decreasing the liver's production of harmful blood fats.

A cautionary note: The scientific community refers to niacin used in megadoses as a drug rather than a vitamin and researchers emphasize that this therapy not be undertaken except under the supervision of a physician. According to *Nutrition and the M.D.*, large doses can cause abnormal liver enzyme levels and heart arrhythmias; they can inhibit the use of free fatty acids as fuel by the heart and they are contraindicated in certain cardiac diseases (November, 1987).

Garlic: It has been reported in several articles that garlic protects against heart disease (and stroke) in the following ways:

1. Lowers blood pressure.
2. Lowers cholesterol levels
3. Decreases triglycerides.
4. Reduces the oxidation of LDL cholesterol.
5. Reduces the tendency of blood to clot.

Earl Mindell reports in his book, *The Miracle Nutrient*, that German researches have found that a substance (called a phytochemical) in garlic inhibits the formation of a hormone which normally raises blood pressure. Levels are also normalized in people with low blood pressure.

Garlic also helps keep the blood from clotting. The *Journal of Orthomolecular Medicine*, March, 1985, states the following: "The amount of platelet aggregation decreased significantly during garlic administration."

Vitamin E: Years ago Drs. Wilfrid and Evan Shute had great clinical success using the vitamin with their heart patients and concluded that it had the following beneficial properties: improves oxygen supply by protecting red blood cells, works as an anti-clotting agent, prevents undesirable excessive scarring of the heart following an infarct, (this is an event instigated by a clot in a coronary artery which causes tissue death in the heart due to reduced oxygen supply), is a vasodilator and improves capillary permeability.

Siri Khalsa reports in *Nutrition News*, 1989 Vol. XII, No. 4, the following: "Current research shows that the level of HDLs in the blood may be increased by vitamin E supplementation."

The highest food form is wheatgerm oil. It is also found in salad oils, almonds, peanuts and seeds, asparagus, mangoes, green leafy vegetables, and wheat germ cereal.

Coenzyme Q_{10}:

CoQ_{10} is a coenzyme necessary for cell respiration, electron transfer and the control of oxidation reactions. It is essential to the health of all tissues and organs in the body. It is an essential catalyst nutrient for cellular energy in the body that declines with age. It has been successful in combating angina and degenerative heart function, and is crucial in the prevention and treatment of congestive heart and arterial diseases. It also reduces high blood pressure without other medication. Although it was initially isolated and researched by American scientists, it was developed as a pharmaceutical product in Japan, where millions have used it for congestive heart failure.

Karl Folkers, Ph.D., Director of the Institute for Biomedical Research at the University of Texas in Austin, is recognized as the world's leader of CoQ_{10} research. For his contributions in this field, his work on vitamins B6 and B12 and other biomedical research, Dr. Folkers was awarded the 1986 Priestley Medal, the highest award of the American Chemical Society.

"In his Priestley Medal address, Dr. Folkers cited examples of dramatic effects heart patients had experienced with therapeutic CoQ_{10} use. One 66-year old man, hospitalized three times in the two years prior to receiving CoQ_{10}, after four years of CoQ_{10} therapy plays golf, mows his lawn and walks two miles daily . . . Twice hospitalized previously for congestive heart failure, an 84-year old woman four years into CoQ_{10} treatment shops, swims, has made two trips to Africa in the second and fourth years of treatment, spends winters in Florida and attends board meetings.

"Dr. Folkers believes that a deficiency of CoQ_{10} is frequently a causative factor of congestive heart failure. He recommends correction of this deficiency with 30-100 mg per day of CoQ_{10} taken orally. The worse the deficiency, the more quickly the person will respond; however, in most cases the response may be slower, taking weeks or several months, because of CoQ_{10}'s vitamin-like action.

"Besides increasing the strength of the heart, CoQ_{10} protects against heart attack, relieves angina, lowers high blood pressure, boosts the immune system, is an effective antioxidant and is a potent weapon against periodontal disease." [1]

Good food sources of this nutrient are mackerel and sardines, cereal brans, wheat germ, beans, nuts, fish, eggs, peanuts, dark green vegetables (like broccoli and spinach), soybeans, soy, sesame and canola oils. The body's ability to assimilate food source CoQ_{10} declines with age. Supplementation has a long history of effectiveness in boosting immunity, increasing cardiac strength, reversing high blood pressure, promoting natural weight loss, and inhibiting aging.

People who are overweight also run a higher risk of heart attacks. The Associated Press gives a new look at the weight the government allows for healthy hearts. Harvard researches say that new findings from a study of more than 115,000 nurses strongly indicate that U.S. weight guidelines are too lax and encourage obesity in both men and women.

Quoting from the Associated Press, "We found that about 40 per cent of all heart attacks that occur in middle-aged women are due to overweight," said Dr. JoAnn E. Manson, co-director of women's health at Harvard-affiliated Brigham and Women's Hospital in Boston. She said similar results are found in men.

The study showed that women of average weight had about a 50 percent higher risk of heart attack than women who were 15 percent less than average U.S. weights. In addition women who gained 10 or fewer pounds in early to middle adulthood had the lowest risk of heart attacks, the researchers reported in today's issue of The Journal of the American Medical Association.

For instance, a 5-foot-6-inch woman had the lowest risk if she weighed less than 130 pounds. At the same height, a weight of 130 to 142 pounds carried 20 percent higher risk. At 142-155 pounds, it was 50 percent higher; at 155 to 180 pounds, it was double.

Regular exercise can fight against heart disease, high cholesterol levels, high blood pressure, overweight, stress, osteoporosis, and constipation. Regular exercise is defined as a minimum of three 20 minute periods of activity per week which raise the heart rate to at least 65 percent of its capacity.

Hawthorn is used primarily as a cardiac tonic and considered valuable for improvement of cardiac weakness, angina pectoris, valve murmurs from heart valve defects, an enlarged heart, sighing respiration, nerve depression or unexplained chronic fatigue.

Scientists have discovered that Hawthorn increases coronary blood flow and improves myocardial metabolism allowing the heart to function with less oxygen. Hawthorn dilates blood vessels, allowing blood to flow more freely and thus, is effective at lowering blood pressure. In addition, it acts directly on the heart muscle to help a damaged heart work more efficiently. Studies have shown that Hawthorn is excellent for both the prevention and treatment of coronary heart disease when used on a regular basis.

Chapter 15

Super Foods

There are many charts, booklets, and guides to help one determine the better foods for the body. One in particular that I like was made available from the Rodale Food Guide. They summed up their idea by making a *target*, the better foods in the bull's eye.

The foods in the *center* of the target are extraordinarily high in vitamins, minerals and other valuable nutrients. Most are rich in fiber and low in fat. They are the following:

Whole Grain foods
Beans
Broccoli
Parsley
Oats
Garbanzo Beans
Lima Beans

Mustard Greens
Turnip Greens
Lentils
Peas
Kidney Beans
Tofu
Kale
Collards
Bran
Sweet Potatoes
Brown Rice
Sprouts
Amaranth greens and grains
Low fat fish which include: cod, flounder, haddock, halibut, perch, pollock, rockfish, sole, catfish
Soybeans
Garlic

The foods in the *next ring* are also excellent, and together with those in the center should make up the bulk of your diet. Most of these foods are quite reasonable in cost. They are the following:

Tomatoes
Watercress
Strawberries
Apricots
Corn
Green Peppers
Oranges

White Potatoes
Bananas
Winter Squash
Papayas
Cabbage
Cantaloupes
Cucumber
Pink Grapefruit
Sunflower Seeds
Spinach
Brussels sprouts
Buttermilk and skim milk
Nectarines
Cauliflower
Peaches
Low-fat yogurt
Nuts (no added salt, sugar or oil)
Chicken and Turkey (without skin)
Carrots
Onions
Tempeh
Herb Teas
Beet Greens
Mushrooms

The foods in the third ring are good and basically healthful, but are third from the top of the list. They are the following:

Peanut butter (no added salt, sugar or oil–freshly ground is the best)
Watermelon
Fatty fish (herring, mackerel, salmon, sardines, and albacore tuna)
Cherries
Rhubarb
Eggs
Celery
Whole milk
Pears
Less fatty cuts of lamb
Cottage Cheese
Less fatty cuts of beef
Apples
Dried fruits
Turnips
Avocado
Veal
Eggplant
Granola
Pineapple
Whole milk yogurt
White grapefruit
Unsweetened fruit juices
Artichokes
Unsalted vegetable juices

The fourth ring are of doubtful healthfulness, mostly because of excessive fat. They are the following:

Most cheese (too salty and high in fat)
Sour Cream
Pizza
Oysters
Cream
Canned Juices and vegetables
Fatty meats
Salad oils
Lobster
Clams
Deep fried poultry and fish
Scallops
Sausage
Margarine

The Rodale Food Guide lists the fifth circle, the one farthest from the bull's eye, as being the one to be avoided, as most contain high amounts of sugar, and saturated fat. They are the following:

Chocolate
Ice Cream
Sugar
Salt
Pickles
Pretzels

Potato Chips
Pudding mixes
Salted snacks
White flour
Soft Drinks
Candy Bars
Soup Mixes
Frankfurters
Sugared Cereals

Chapter 16

Wonder Foods

Wonder foods does not mean that they can produce miracles; the term merely indicates that, ounce for ounce, these special foods contain more repair materials than others. Linda Clark says in her book, *Secrets of Health and Beauty,* that "People who use them report quicker health benefits than from eating ordinary foods. Since they contain a higher-than-average amount of vitamins and minerals and are surprisingly inexpensive, they are an excellent value... What are these wonder foods? They include liver, brewers yeast, rice polishings, blackstrap, wheat germ, yogurt, lecithin, various seeds and oils." [1]   I must also add, aloe vera juice and gel to this list.

Aloe Vera Juice and Gel

Aloe is rich in *vitamin C*, which helps maintain good blood vessel tone and aids in promoting healthy circulation.

Potassium in Aloe aids the heart's rhythm and stimulates the kidney to dispose of body wastes, thus making Aloe a natural cleanser.

Calcium in Aloe, participates in clotting, activates enzymes that are helpful for proper digestion, regulates the passage of fluids through cellular walls and works to regulate the contraction and relaxation of the heart muscle.

Sodium in the leaves, combined with the potassium, helps maintain a favorable acid base and normal water-level balance.

Manganese in Aloe, is needed for maximum efficiency of certain food-digesting enzymes; it also helps build resistance to disease and helps deter kidney stones.

Magnesium in Aloe gel helps protect against kidney stones and has been used to treat severe angina and coronary thrombosis.

Silicon in Aloe gel joins with other minerals to create tooth enamel and build strong bones.

Iron in Aloe gel carries oxygen to the brain, and is needed to form good red blood cells.

Copper in Aloe gel is present to help convert iron in hemoglobin.

Aloe also accomplishes the following:

1. Aloe also has the ability to penetrate tissue, break down and digest dead tissue through the action of its enzymes, and enhance normal cell proliferation.

2. Because of its extraordinary penetrating power, Aloe is able to relieve pain deep within the joints and muscles.

3. Aloe Vera inhibits the growth of several kinds of harmful bacteria, including staphylococcus and salmonella.

4. The Food and Drug Administration, a conservative organization at best, conceded that Aloe Vera actually accelerated the regeneration of damaged skin tissue, internally and externally.

5. As a vegetable drink, Aloe Vera is purported to reduce the flow of stomach acid and to soothe upset stomachs.

6. Regular use of Aloe Vera juice can help maintain regularity, minimize fatigue, maximize endurance, promote proper digestion, replace electrolytes (preventing muscle cramps) and help keep the body's system in proper balance.

Aloe Vera Gel is one of the finest body cleansers and brings most gratifying results. It cleans the morbid matter from the stomach, liver, kidneys, spleen and bladder and is the finest colon cleanser known. In turn, this process purifies the blood.

Aloe Vera Gel is also rich in Amino Acids, which are chains of atoms constructing protein in the body, and Enzymes, which rejuvenate aged tissue and promote healthy skin.

Yeast

There are several kinds of yeast: brewers, torula, and yeast mixes. brewer's yeast is one of the greatest sources of B vitamins, minerals and protein. Brewer's yeast contains about ten times as much protein as the same amount of whole-wheat flour. It is extraordinarily rich in Nucleic Acid, which is a basic element in cell development and is believed to retard the aging process. It is the best nutritional source of Chromium, which occurs in brewer's yeast in an organic compound known as GTF (Glucose Tolerance Factor). This vital factor is essential for the production of functionally effective insulin, without which the body cannot properly handle glucose-its major fuel.

It contains the following:

Vitamins:
B-1
B-2
B-6
Niacin
Choline
Inositol
Panthothenic acid
Para-amino-benzoic acid (PABA)
Biotin
Folic Acid

Amino Acids:
Lysine
Tryptophane
Histidine
Phenylalanine
Leucine
Methionine
Valine
Glycine
Alanine
Aspartic Acid
Glutamic acid
Proline
Hydroxproline
Tyrosine
Cystine
Arginine

Minerals:
Phosphorus
Potassium
Magnesium
Silicon
Calcium
Copper
Manganese
Zinc
Aluminum
Sodium
Iron

Tin
Boron
Gold
Silver
Nickel
Cobalt
Iodine

One heaping tablespoon of *Yeast 500 Plus Vitamins* includes the following:

Calories	50
Protein	5.5 grams
Carbohydrates	7.2 grams
Fat	0
Sodium	135 mg
Potassium	320 mg
Vitamin B1	8 mg
Vitamin B2	8 mg
Niacin	40 mg
Calcium	375 mg
Iron	5 mg
Vitamin B6	8 mg
Folic Acid	100 mcg
Vitamin B12	12 mcg
Phosphorous	376 mg
Iodine	0.1 mg
Magnesium	150 mg
Zinc	2 mg
Copper	0.28 mg
Biotin	25 mcg

Pantothenic Acid	32 mg
Choline	88 mg
Manganese	0.56 mg
Sodium	135 mg

Approximate Amino Acids per heaping tablespoon:

Alanne	435 mg
Arginine	286 mg
Aspartic Acid	620 mg
Glutamic Acid	1009 mg
Glycine	278 mg
Histidine	168 mg
Isoleucine	277 mg
Cysteine	85 mg
Hydoxypoline	240 mg
Leucine	434 mg
Lysine	450 mg
Methionine	87 mg
Phenylalanine	240 mg
Proline	264 mg
Threonine	277 mg
Serinne	270 mg
Tryptophan	58 mg
Tyrosine	260 mg
Valine	357 mg

Adelle Davis lists some findings of the value of nutritional yeast in her book, *Let's Get Well*. They are as follows:

- If the inositol and choline (both B vitamins) content is high, together with liver, wheat germ and lecithin, yeast helps to lower cholesterol.
- In one study, two tablespoons of yeast daily plus a multivitamin capsule, produced a rapid improvement in all 68 people suffering from cirrhosis of the liver. As long as the diet continued, there was no return of liver damage.
- Cases of eczema (also acne) often clear up quickly with nutritional yeast.
- Yeast has greatly increased survival of rats given cancer causing substances.
- The ache and stabbing pains of neuritis are helped with yeast and liver.

A woman writing in *Prevention* magazine, December 1958, stated, "My husband developed a severe pain in his left jaw. It persisted for days, becoming unbearable . . . A doctor diagnosed it as *tic douloureux* and knew of no relief for the pain except surgery and morphine . . . This disease is an inflammation of the fifth nerve of the face. I thought, what is good for nerves? Vitamin B. What is the best source of vitamin B? Brewers yeast.

"That night my husband took two tablespoons of yeast and has taken that amount ever since. The results have been almost magic. The pain gradually left. At the end of two weeks it was completely gone and has never returned."

The best way to take brewers yeast is to stir one to three heaping tablespoons into fruit juice and swallow quickly (start with smaller portions). *Lewis Laboratories' Imported Brewer's Yeast* has the best tasting brewer's yeast.

Yogurt

Yogurt has been used for centuries in many countries. The major value of yogurt is that it helps the intestinal tract. Yogurt is also a natural antibiotic. Noted nutrition expert Linda Clark reports, "Studies have shown that an 8 ounce jar, refrigerated for seven days, provides an antibiotic value equal to 14 penicillin units" [2]

"Henry Seneca, M.D., has reported studies in a medical journal showing that yogurt kills amoeba in five minutes; typhus, *S. paratyphus, Br. abortus V. comma, B, subtillis teriae, P. vulgaris, M. pyogenes.* In five hours it kills *E. coll, K. pneumonia,* streptococcus, and staphylococcus. In twenty-four hours it kills *L. lactic, C. diphtheriae, S. mitis,* and *S. fecallis.* Other bacteria too numerous to mention are also destroyed by yogurt. Unlike an antibiotic drug, however, yogurt does away with only the disturbing bacteria, without killing the beneficial bacteria. Truly a wonder food!" [3]

Yogurt contains protein as well as calcium and sufficient acid to help digest both. Yogurt is a kind of predigested protein. It is 91% digested after one hour, while milk is only 32% digested in the same time. Yogurt aids the body to manufacture B vitamins. It is also helpful in relieving constipation.

For this use take one cup of yogurt per day. (This is the natural yogurt, not mixed with sugar).

There are many ways to use yogurt. You can mix a little fruit and honey with it and make a good dessert. You can use it as a substitute for sour cream, and it can be used on baked potatoes with chives and in salad dressings. It should never be cooked, since cooking destroys its active, friendly bacteria.

Liver

Liver probably contains more nutritional values than any other single food. It is a rich source of vitamins, minerals, and easily assimilated protein. It also contains a rich supply of vitamin B-12. Many people do not like the taste of liver and because of the possibility of less-than-the-best liver supply, it can be taken in tablet form.

Liver contains calcium, phosphorus, vitamins A, B1, B2 Niotinic acid, B12, and C, and is considered a brain food. Morton S. Biskind, M.D., considers liver, in addition to vitamins, a necessity for regaining health. He says, "Simply adding desiccated liver or suitable liver fractions to the regime invariably has resulted in a lasting improvement, often evident within a few days." [4]

Linda Clark says that liver is useful for beauty also. A woman with gorgeous hair and skin told her, "I eat lots of liver. It feeds and nourishes my skin and hair from the inside. Before I learned this beauty secret my skin and hair were drab." She took 30 tablets of desiccated liver daily.

Blackstrap molasses

Raw sugar cane is rich in vitamins and minerals. Those who eat this natural product are reported not to develop tooth decay. After the sap from sugar cane has been collected, three different products are extracted from it. The third and final extraction is blackstrap molasses, the nutritionally richest of all three extractions. It is one of the foods highest in iron. (Iron in one tablespoon of blackstrap is the equivalent to that in nine eggs.) Blackstrap is richer in copper than most foods. It is an excellent source of B vitamins, and contains one of the highest levels of the mineral potassium to be found in any food. It contains more calcium than milk. The following analysis of blackstrap molasses is from the *Journal of the American Medical Association* (July 14, 1951):

Analysis of Blackstrap Molasses
Five tablespoons of blackstrap molasses contains:

Minerals:

Calcium	258 mg.
Phosphorus	30 mg.
Iron	7.97 mg.
Copper	1.93 mg.
Potassium	1500 mg.

B vitamins:

Inositol	150 mg.
Thiamin	245 mg.

Riboflavin	240 mg.
Niacin	4 mg.
Pyridoxine	270 mg.
Pantothenic acid	260 mg.
Biotin	16 mg.

The benefits of blackstrap are many. It is a good laxative. Because it contains large amounts of inositol, it is credited with stopping falling hair. Because of its high potassium content, it is a valuable aid for hearts. It is beneficial to those who suffer with anemia.

Each morning you can put two tablespoons of blackstrap in a cup of hot water with lemon and drink to your health. You can also add a little to your homemade brown gravies (gives color, taste and nutritional value). Some people add it to their teas, while others drink it in a nutritional milkshake.

Chapter 17

Walk and Exercise Your Way to Health

The testimonies below appeared in the August, 1993 Magazine, *Walking*. Geralyn B. Simandl was diagnosed with multiple sclerosis in 1990. She responded to this diagnosis by taking up fitness walking. "Ironically, the first things the M.S. affected were my legs and my ability to walk," says Simandl. "I was devastated, but I realized it was time to do everything in my power to keep this disease at bay." For Simandl, 36, this meant losing weight and increasing her endurance and muscle strength. She went on a low-fat diet and began walking one mile two to three times a week on a straight farm road near her home in Delavan, Wisconsin. Gradually, she worked her way up to 12 miles a week.

In March 1992, Simandl reached her 75-pound weight-loss goal, and her disease went into remission. "My life has changed dramatically because of my new approach to fitness," says Simandl, who started her own catering business and went back to school full time. "It's unfortunate that it took a disease to wake me up to the importance of good health, but the point is that I did, and I am able to relish and reap the benefits of that discovery."

Gary Ricci who weighed 360 pounds, said, "I've been on every diet imaginable, but it wasn't until I began a daily walking program that the weight started coming off and staying off." As a reminder of his former weight problem Gary keeps hanging on the wall in front of his treadmill: a pair of pants he wore when he weighed 360 pounds, and the belt that held them up around his 56-inch waist.

"I went on a low-fat diet and started out slowly–walking 5 to 10 minutes every day. Then I began walking farther and farther," says Ricci, who was up to 5.5 mile walks near his home in West Peabody, Mass, in 1993. "Walking has almost become an obsession because of the way it makes me feel," he says. "I believe the feeling of euphoria I get is the same as the runner's high."

Dr. James Hutchinson started walking 6 to 8 miles a day near his office in San Mateo, California. "I always say walking is an inexpensive way to discard the bitter baggage and all the real or imagined hurts of your life," says Hutchinson. He says that walking has helped him relieve stress. Hutchinson prescribes walking to most of his patients, no matter what their condition.

Seventy two-year-old Louis Harris, the noted pollster and public-opinion analyst, and author of six books, wrote an article entitled, "Heal Thyself," printed in the 1996 April *Reader's Digest*.

One day he discovered he could not walk over two city blocks before his feet tingled and grew numb and his legs cramped up with the excruciating pain. He went to Dr. Gary Giangola, a vascular surgeon at New York University Medical Center in New York City. His diagnosis was occlusions in the femoral arteries in both legs, caused by a buildup of plaque that extends all the way up to the aorta. Dr. Giangola explained that he could operate on his diseased arteries, but the surgery would be dangerous and expensive. "You know," he said, "you're in pretty good shape for your age. If you'll walk at least a mile every day, I think your body will cure the clogged-artery problem by itself."

In disbelief, Louis asked Dr. Giangola how he could do that. "When you walk day after day," he answered, "your muscles send out signals for more blood flow. Very slowly, over time, your body responds by making new arteries called collaterals. These collaterals bypass the blocked arteries just as surgery would. Walking is the key—other exercises won't do it, because they don't provide adequate stimulation for the collaterals to grow."

Louis told the doctor he could not walk two blocks, much less a mile. Dr. Giangola told him to stop every two blocks, wait a couple of minutes and start again when his muscles had recovered. Seven months after he was first stricken, Louis became very depressed, called the doctor, and told him he would just have surgery instead. At his scheduled appointment with the doctor, he was left in the waiting room for over two hours, in which time he saw a parade of people, some missing legs, some in wheelchairs, others struggling to stand. When he finally got to see the doctor, he told him his waiting room looked like a Civil War emergency room.

"That was exactly what I wanted you to see," Dr. Giangola answered. "Now get back to walking."

Louis now walks three to four miles every day, has stopped eating fatty foods, and eats fish, poultry, raw vegetables and fresh fruit.

Gayelord Hauser writes the following in his book, *New Treasury of Secrets*, "A New York physician said bluntly that half the patients in his waiting room could cure themselves of what ailed them if they would spend an hour walking every day. Walking cures tensions, insomnia, chronic fatigue, and a host of minor physical and mental complaints that drag down the spirit and body and take the joy out of living. Walking, free striding, free-swinging, rhythmic, brisk but unhurried walking, is the perfect aid to digestion, elimination, circulation, relaxation of body, mind, and spirit." [1]

Chapter 18

The Amazing Aminos

There are twenty-two amino acids known to be necessary to the proper functioning of the human body. They combine with nitrogen to form thousands of different proteins as the letters of the alphabet combine to form thousands of different words.

Protein, the only food group containing nitrogen, is broken down by the digestive system. The resulting amino acids and nitrogen are carried throughout the body by the bloodstream. Needy cells attract the amino acids and nitrogen they require to reproduce, building new protein substances for the body such as tissues, hormones and enzymes. Because they are used to form new proteins, the amino acids are often called *the building blocks of the body*.

Amino acids are not interchangeable. Each one has a specific function. The body cannot make, maintain, or repair a particular protein unless each individual amino acid necessary for that protein is available. In studies that have been completed with essential amino acids, it has been found that elimination of just one resulted in a negative nitrogen balance with symptoms such as appetite failure, nervous irritability and a sensation of extreme fatigue. The symptoms disappeared as soon as the missing amino acid was restored to the diet.

Of the 22 known amino acids, fourteen can be manufactured by the cells from fat or sugar combined with the nitrogen freed from the breakdown of digested proteins. The other eight must be supplied. These eight are called essential amino acids, EAA's.

Although the 22 amino acids work together to rebuild and repair the body, research has shown that individual amino acids have a phenomenal positive effect on our physical and mental health. These "amazing aminos" include *l-tryptophank l-glutamine, and l-lysine.*

L-tryptophan alleviates stress, anxiety, depression and insomnia. Also available knowledge indicates that l-tryptophan is extremely valuable to heart health. Dr. O. Norman Shealy, stress expert and neurosurgeon say, "L-tryptophan is terrific. It can let you throw away your tranquilizers, sleeping pills, and dangerous anti-depressant drugs forever."

In the *Waking and Sleeping Journal 1,* Dr. Ernest Hartman, Boston State Hospital and Tufts University School of Medicine, reported that one gram of l-tryptophan given 20 minutes before retiring, cut in half the time necessary for falling to sleep.

L-tryptophan is the least abundant amino acid in most tissues and foods. It is found in many high protein foods such as milk, yogurt, cheese, fish, chicken, meats, beans, peas, eggs and peanuts. However, getting large amounts of l-trytophan through foods is almost impossible. Dr. Shealy recommends that l-tryptophan be taken twice daily in times of special stress. Since l-tryptophan will not be used properly by the body if there is a deficiency of B6, it is a good idea to accompany it with a B-complex supplement.

Tryptophan is generally known because of its role in alleviating insomnia, stress, anxiety, and depression, but it is also valuable to heart health.

Dr. Pamela Bryne of Stockton, has advised me that tryptophan can only be attained through prescription now. However, there is something else that can be taken without prescription, that works quite well: Melatonin. As already discussed elsewhere in this book, "Melatonin is the primary messenger of the pineal gland, and through melatonin the pineal performs its many jobs. Melatonin is not the only compound found in the pineal gland. Melatonin is actually synthesized from two other compounds: tryptophan, an amino acid, and serotonin, another neurotransmitter. Melatonin is produced from these compounds as the body needs it." [1]

One of the best known of the free form amino acids is L-lysiene. It is an essential amino acid. (Remember, this means the body cannot make l-lysine from fats or sugar and free nitrogen, you must supply it.) It is the most inhibiting on the growth of viruses. It was introduced to the public in the late 1970's as a remedy for reducing the severity and incidence of herpes infections. Used along with vitamins C and A and the minerals zinc and calcium (lysiene is necessary for calcium absorption), it can suppress and prevent viral growth by improving the body's nutrient balance. Lysine is abundant in soy, meat and dairy products; it is low in many vegetable, grain and seed proteins.

Lysiene also plays an important part in the production of hormones, enzymes and antibodies as well as in tissue repair and tissue growth. I have found it to be an excellent way to treat mouth or canker sores. Take several capsules of lysiene throughout the day when you first feel the discomforting pain of these little white sores, and they will disappear very quickly.

L-glutamine has been called a "natural wonder." Actually glutamine is not an amino acid at all but a precursor to the amino acid glutamic acid. Glutamic acid has the unique property of being one of only two substance which provide fuel for the brain. (The other one is glucose: blood sugar.)

Although glutamic acid is the amino acid which the brain uses, studies show that it does not cross the brain barrier as readily as does glutamine.

According to Richard Passwater, Ph.D., " . . . large amounts of glutamic acid produce only a trivial elevation of glutamic acid in the brain, [while] moderate amounts of L-glutamine produce marked elevation..."

Glutamic acid promotes improved mental alertness and memory. Throughout the body, glutamic acid serves as a buffer against the accrual of excess ammonia. A shortage of glutamine in the diet or of glutamic acid in the brain results, at worst, in brain damage due to excess ammonia, or, at best, in a brain that just never gets into high gear.

Because of its ability to repair and regenerate the membrane of the digestive organs, it has been very effective in the treatment of peptic ulcers. In 1957, Dr. William Shive of the University of Texas did some pioneer research with excellent results when he successfully isolated l-glutamine from cabbage juice (a food long recommended by Dr. Airola for effectiveness in dealing with ulcers). L-glutamine actually helps the body to avoid a relapse of the ulcers by reducing and clearing niches on the digestive membrane.

Dr. H.L. Newbold, *Mega-Nutrients for Your Nerves*, recommends l-glutamine to fight fatigue, depression, and impotence.

Dr. Robert Williams, the famous biochemist who discovered both vitamins B6 and B10, has been writing about glutamine since 1959. He recommends 1-4 grams daily in divided doses. It is also tasteless so it can be mixed with food or water without detection.

All the amino acids will be more effective if taken along with full spectrum amino acid capsules as well as with vitamins B6 and C, which assist the action of the aminos in the body.

Chapter 19

Powerful Herbs

Garlic: Researchers James A. North and Byron K. Murray, two microbiologists at Bringham Young University, in 1989 concluded that garlic extract can destroy certain viruses, including those which cause fever blisters, smallpox, and genital herpes. "Historically, garlic has been used for medicinal purposes," Murray said. "We are reporting that garlic extract inactivates certain viruses and that it kills these viruses 99.9 percent of the time."

Allicin,* the flavor substance in garlic, is converted in the body to a drug very much like Mucodyne (S-carboxymethylcysteine), prescribed in Europe for lung problems. Garlic's abilities to relieve chest congestion have been recognized almost as long as mankind has been eating "the stinking rose," as it is sometimes called.

219

*Dr. Earl Mindell says that onions, radishes and leeks also contain *allicin,* which can destroy disease germs without sweeping away the friendly bacteria in the process.

Garlic is a cholesterol-lowering, antibiotic, anti-cancer, and anti-pollutant natural substance. Nutrition News says, "Perhaps its major attribute is its ability to decrease platelet aggregation (sticky blood), lowering the risk of heart attack in much the same way as aspirin without aspirin's possible side effects of low level gastrointestinal bleeding and peptic ulceration. It is also helpful for normalizing blood pressure.

Siri Khalsa, reports in *Nutrition News, 1995 Volume XIX, No. 11,* that Garlic protects against heart disease (and stroke) in these ways:

1. Lowers blood pressure
2. Lowers cholesterol levels
3. Decreases triglycerides
4. Reduces the tendency of blood to clot
5. Reduces the oxidation of LDL cholesterol

Garlic's ability to lower blood pressure was reported as early as 1948 by a Swiss physician at the university of Geneva. Dr. F.G. Piotrowsky administered garlic to 100 patients with hypertension and found that garlic lowered blood pressure in 40 of them.

Jean Carper, author of *Food: Your Miracle Medicine*, says that garlic is sometimes called

"Russian Penicillin." When nothing can cure a cold, many people believe that eating a couple of peeled raw cloves of garlic will head off a cold.

Ginseng is called the "King of Herbs" in the Orient, and has a strengthening and revitalizing effect on the brain, nerve and glandular functions. Ginseng is a stress reducer and gives energy and calmness simultaneously. The restorative and normalizing properties of ginseng have been shown to be useful in the treatment of the three major degenerative diseases: diabetes, heart disease, and cancer.

Echinacea has long been used in North America and originally was used by the people of the Plain's tribes. It is known as a supreme immune enhancer, and is frequently used for colds and flu. It works by stimulating white blood cell production. It also has anti-inflammatory action and is a blood and lymphatic purifier.

Ginkgo is one of the world's oldest living plants. The leaves of the ginkgo tree affect the entire vascular system. It is especially famous for its ability to boost the flow of blood to the brain, increasing alertness. It is being researched for possible use in the treatment of Alzheimer's.

Chamomile is most famous as a soothing tea and a remedy for children's complaints. It is useful as a mild sedative. Developed in Europe as a cosmetic for both hair and skin, it contains the active ingredient levomenol that is said to moisturize dry skin and hair. It helps soothe nerves, muscle pain, and helps alleviate insomnia.

Astragalus is a well-known Oriental herb. It is known as a potent immune enhancer. Rob McCaleb, president and founder of the Herb Research Foundation, refers to recent research that indicates its ability to restore the function of damaged immune cells removed from cancer patients. Jeff Kronick, president of Auro Trading Company, a well-known natural products distributing company, and the formulator of the acclaimed line of herbal products Alive Energy Products, said, "Astragalas is unsurpassed at increasing overall systematic energy.

St. John's Wort, for hundreds of years believed to be a magic protector, now is known to be a potent herbal antioxidant. Because of its super high broad spectrum flavonoid content, it protects the body from the damaging and aging effects of metabolic oxidation. St. John's Wort is one of the most useful for the nervous system, effective for the treatment of neuralgia, nerve pains, and injuries as well as for mild depression. It is also used to treat urinary tract problems, and in Europe, extracts have been used as a remedy for bed wetting.

Dandelion is renowned for its effects on the liver, skin, and blood. The green leaves of the dandelion are rich in both beta carotene and potassium. Their nutrition is easily integrated into salads when the leaves are fresh and young. The roots are an excellent diuretic and tonic. The root and leaves together are excellent for the liver and kidneys. One herbalist exclaimed, "The dandelion is an herbal pharmacy in itself!"

Dong Quai is the most famous of all women's herbs. It produces a calm, relaxed energy for women. It is used to regulate the menses, to increase fertility and to stabilize the process of menopause.

Rosemary has been used for headaches, depression, and muscle spasms. It has been recommended by some herbalists to combine rosemary with gotu kola, ginseng and ginkgo to increase oxygen to the brain and improve memory.

Nettles is a very nutritious herb, high in A, C, iron, and protein. It strengthens the kidneys, stimulates mothers' milk, and increases the body's utilization of oxygen. Leaves gathered before the plant flowers and made into a tea are said to bring relief from asthma.

Milk thistle is recommended for the liver and spleen. It has been known to help restore good digestion and clear up food allergies after bouts with hepatitis.

Alfalfa contains all vitamins/minerals known to man. Alfalfa will help overacidity, the pituitary gland, arthritis, is highly nutritious and will alkalize the body and detoxify the liver.

The herbs and other healthy foods eaten by the people of the Holy Land in biblical times were cited by the Roman historian Tacitus as one reason the Israelites were noted for both their vigor and glowing good health. Historian Henri Daniel-Rops listed the following 16 herbs that were used by the Israelites to stay healthy and energetic in his book, *Palestine in the Time of Jesus.*

1.   **Aloe**: Mentioned frequently in the pages of the Bible, this cactus-like plant can heal, rejuvenate, and energize the body inside and out. So valuable was this rejuvenating plant in the Holy Land that in the Book of Numbers, Balaam praised the Israelites by comparing them to "aloe planted by the Lord" (Numbers 24:6).

2.   **Coriander**: This valuable herb helps keep the heart healthy, soothes bowel problems, and acts as a stimulant to restore appetite and vigor.

3.   **Horseradish**: This was one of the bitter herbs eaten at Passover meals. This ancient root dissolves the fat in the cells, invigorates the body by cleansing it of harmful toxins, and is known as a potent diuretic that flushes away excess fluids and purifies the kidneys.

4.   **Hyssop**: In biblical times, hyssop tea was used as a tranquilizer. Herbalists recommend the tea for reducing stress caused high blood pressure.

5.   **Saffron**: Saffron induces sweating, which rejuvenates the body by removing toxins, and will flush out gas from the stomach and intestines.

6.   **Dill**: Herbalists recommend dill to calm jumpy stomachs and keep the heart healthy.

7.   **Anise**: This spicy herb mentioned in the Bible is a known remedy for lung problems and coughing.

This licorice-flavored herb also eases digestion caused by nervousness.

8. **Marjoram**: A part of the everyday diet in biblical times, this tasty herb served as a tea is an excellent energy-giving tonic.

9. **Rosemary**: One of the herbs the people of Israel used to season their food, rosemary improves circulation, memory, digestion, and reduces high blood pressure.

10. **Parsley**: Parsley was included in the everyday diet of the Israelites. This leafy herb improves skin appearance, prevents kidney and bladder problems, is a natural diuretic, and freshens bad breath.

11. **Chamomile**: This was used in biblical times to flavor food and as a tea to calm jangled nerves. It is also known as a heart toner.

12. **Garlic**: A staple in the diet of all the ancient peoples, this pungent herb was valued by the Israelites who recognized its incredible healing powers. Modern medical research has shown garlic to be a powerful antibiotic and a blood cleanser which rids the body of harmful cholesterol. It can even be effective in preventing some forms of cancer, studies have shown.

13. **Mustard**: Mentioned in both the Old and New Testaments, this tiny seed helps remove harmful substances from fatty foods, and it relieves arthritis and rheumatism pain when added to bath water.

14. **Mint**: Mint tea keeps the body cool in hot weather and has a calming effect on the nerves.

15.   **Comfrey**:   It has been called a wonder herb that is effective as a remedy for most health problems.   It was in use 3,000 years ago to flush toxins from the body.

16.   **Cumin**:   Cumin is a tonic and heart strengthener.

Chapter 20

&motional &ealth

&utritional health cannot be separated from emotional health; they are entertwined together. Every person has four areas which they must work on or be aware of their particular needs: spiritual, emotional, physical, and social. To be truly healthy these four facets of the personality must be held in balance.

The attitude with which a person faces a particular situation will also affect the health of that individual. From the writings of the Old Testament it is proven over and over that the tongue and attitudes affect the heart, countenance and even the bones. Those truths are as follows:

- As a man thinketh in his heart so is he (Proverbs 23:7).
- The tongue of the wise is health (Proverbs 12:18).

- A trusting heart shall bring health to the navel and marrow to the bones (Proverbs 3:5-8).

Bone is the framework of the body, and is one of the most active tissues of the body. It cleanses the blood of harmful substances. It stores useful materials such as calcium, fluoride, phosphorus and sodium. Bone also contains red bone marrow where new red blood cells are made. It is a network of blood cells, connective tissue, and blood-forming cells. About two-thirds of the weight of bony tissue is mineral matter, chiefly calcium and phosphorus. The rest is organic matter, consisting largely of collagen, a fibrous protein.

There are 6 chief causes of death: emotional, nutritional, poisons, infections, accidents, and genetic. The greatest cause of disease is emotional.

Stress can make you sick because of its connection with the immune system. In the book, *The Melatoin Miracle,* Drs. Pierpaoli and William Regelson state that, "Stress can have a devastating effect on the immune system. People who are under physical or mental stress are more vulnerable to disease, and more likely to fall prey to a viral or bacerial infection that, under less stressful circumstances, they might be able to shake off.

"It [stress] not only inflicts emotional suffering, but can lead to physical damage. According to the American Academy of Family Physicians, more than two thirds of all visits to the doctor are due to stress-related ailments, which include asthma, anxiety, headache, indigestion, fatigue, and nausea. Worker's compensation claims for stress-related ailments have increased 700 percent over the past decade. Numerous studies have documented the link between severe stress and gastrointestinal problems like colitis, heart disease, and even cancer." [1]

In addition to causing headache pain, stress can make it difficult to concentrate and can even impair memory. It can also lead to insomnia, depression, panic attacks, and chronic overeating. Stress can increase heart rate, disturb heart rhythms, cause blood vessels to constrict and reduce the blood flow to the heart. Stress can cause nausea, gastritis, stomach cramps, constipation or diarrhea. It can contract muscles, causing pain and stiffness. The most affected places are in the lower back, neck, knees and hip. Stress can cause hives and eczema, and may increase breathing rate and result in hyperventilation or dizziness. Chronic elevated stress hormones can weaken the body's ability to fight infection, resulting in less resistance to colds, and possibly more serious diseases. Not only does continual stress weaken the immune system, but it is weakened further if accompanied by a negative attitude. Stress can also worsen discomforts of PMS and menopause.

The following suggestions are proven ways to help improve your emotional health and handle stress better:

1. *Change Your Thoughts:*
You are what you think. Facial muscles definitely react to thoughts and emotions. What you are and how you treat people affect your health. "The merciful man doeth good to his own soul; but he that is cruel troubleth his own flesh" (Proverbs 11:17).

Dr. Robert Ornstein writes in his book *Healthy Pleasures*, that optimism may favorably affect our immune function. He told of how comparisons of blood samples from optimists and pessimists revealed a better ration of "helper" to "suppressor" lumphocytes, suggesting that the white blood cells of optimists may be more effective in defending the body against tumors. He shares also that a "study of patients with advanced breast and skin cancer revealed that a joyful attitude and optimistic style were the strongest psychological predictors of how long the patients would remain cancer-free before the disease returned." [2]

2. *Proper Nutrition Helps to Combat Stress*
Billie Jay Sahley, Ph.D., recommends in her clinical practice in San Antonio, Texas, all the B-complex vitamins to fight emotional and physical tension, excessive fatigue, noise, and anxiety. Vitamin C can help to alleviate damage from stress. Dr. Sahley says, "Vitamin C is an antioxidant; it helps to neutralize foreign substances, chemicals and poisons in the body. The body's need for vitamin C

increases greatly during times of any form of stress." ³

She also recommends vitamins A, D and E, calcium, magnesium, potassium, phosphorus, manganese, iron and zinc.

Dr. James Balch recommends in the book, *Prescription for Nutritional Healing,* the following herbs for stress: catnip, chamomile, lady slipper, passionflower, pau d'arco, rose hips, Siberian ginseng, skullcap, and valerian root.

3. *Listen to Good Music:*

An article, "Music's Surprising Power to Heal," written by David M. Mazie, states that music can help a patient to relax, thereby quickening the healing process. He quotes Dr. Clyde L. Nash of St. Luke's Hospital in Cleveland, "Music reduces staff tension in the operating room, and also helps relax the patient." One of his patients, Marianne Strebely, severely injured in an auto accident, while awaiting anesthesia, surrounded by a surgical team, was hooked up to a computer that monitored her heart rate and brain waves. She was also hooked up, by earphones, to a tape recorder playing Vivaldi's *The Four Seasons*, and had this to say about her experience in the hospital. "The music was better than the medication. I remained calm before the operation and didn't need as much sedation."

At Baltimore's St. Agnes Hospital, classical music was provided in the critical-care units. Dr.

Raymond Bahr, head of the coronary-care unit states that, "Half an hour of music produced the same effect as ten milligrams of Valium."

Drs. Ornstein and Sobel state in their book, *Healthy Pleasures,* that "music had an effect comparable to that of an intravenous dose of 2.5 milligrams of Valium." [4] While the two do not agree on the amount, they agree that music has the effect of valium to calm the nerves and reduce the level of stress hormones in the blood.

The right kind of music helps lower blood pressure, basal-metabolism and respiration rates, thus lessening physiological responses to stress. Some studies suggest that music may help increase production of endorphins (natural pain relievers) and S-IgA (salivary immunoglobulin A). S-IgA speeds healing, reduces the danger of infection and controls heart rate.

When you feel your stress level overloaded, or your emotional health threatened, it is time to listen to music that will make you feel good, help you relax, or free you from the level of tense anxiety. Sing more, hum more, feed your mind and spirit with good music, and you will definitely notice a change in your frustrated emotions.

4. *Pray a Prayer to God:*

Willliam Sadler, psychiatrist, advises physicians how to get at the cause of people's troubles. He writes, "Prayer is a powerful and effectual worry-remover. Men and women who have learned to pray with childlike sincerity, literally talking to, and communing with the Heavenly Father, are in possession of the great secret whereby they can cast their care upon God, knowing that He careth for us. A clear conscience is a great step toward barricading the mind against neuroticism."

He continues, "Many are victims of fear and worry because they fail properly to maintain their spiritual nutrition . . . The majority of people liberally feed their bodies, and many make generous provision for their mental nourishment; but the vast majority leave the soul to starve, paying very little attention to their spiritual nutrition; and as a result the spiritual nature is so weakened that it is unable to exercise the restraining influence over the mind which would enable it to surmount its difficulties and maintain an atmosphere above conflict and despondency." [5]

Many times desperate prayers are accompanied with tears. Drs. Orstein and Sobel write in the book, *Healthy Pleasures,* the following: "Tear researcher William Frey contends that emotional crying is an eliminative process in which tears actually remove toxic substances from the body, helping to restore physiological and emotional balance.

"Emotional tears also appear to contain endorphins, ACTH, prolactin, and growth hormone, all of which are released by stress. So crying may 'cleanse the mind' in a much more literal sense than even the catharsis theorists imagined." [6]

What better place to pray, than the church? A medical researcher at John Hopkins University discovered that attending church is good for your health. Dr. George W. Comstock of the university's Department of Epidemiology reported that the risk of fatal heart diseases is almost twice as high for the non-churchgoer than for men who attend once a week or more.

5. *Enjoy and Be Aware of Simple Things:*

Oscar Wilde wrote that "simple pleasures are the last refuge of the complex." They may be the best defense against illness. It is refreshing to enjoy a beautiful sunset, *listen* to the solitude of the forest, watch a robin build her nest, or walk through a quiet walnut orchard at dusk. Simple pleasures surround us, but sometimes we are so rushed and tense, that we are blind to the very things that could help take away the tension.

It is important instead of seeing trees, to look closely at *a* tree. See the intricate pattern of the leaf, smell the fragrance, notice the shape of the branches, observe the bird with the cocked head, sense the steady rhythm of growth, the solid structure of nature, and enjoy the moment. The healing power of nature is everywhere. Open your eyes to it.

6. *Try to Relax! Don't Rush:*

Slow down, go with the flow. The old saying, "The hurrier I go, the behinder I get," is true in many ways. You may get there faster, but in what condition did you arrive? The advice, "Take time to smell the roses," is still good advice today, and will help alleviate frustration and nervous tension.

7. *Learn to Laugh Easily:*

The *Executives' Digest* reports the following: "Scientists have been studying the effect of laughter on human beings and have found, among other things, that laughter has a profound and instantaneous effect on virtually every important organ in the human body. Laughter reduces health-sapping tensions and relaxes the tissues as well as exercising the most vital organs. It is said that laughter, even when forced, results in beneficial effect on us, both mentally and physically. Next time you feel nervous and jittery, indulge in a good laugh.

"Hearty laughter is a genial exercise of the body, a form of 'inner jogging.' A robust laugh gives the muscles of your face, shoulders, diaphragm, and abdomen a good workout. With convulsive and sidesplitting laughter, even your arm and leg muscles come into play. Your heart rate and blood pressure temporarily rise, breathing becomes faster and deeper, and oxygen surges throughout your bloodstream. A vigorous laugh can burn up as many calories per hour as brisk walking or cycling.

"While laughing itself may be arousing, the afterglow of a hearty laugh is positively relaxing. Blood pressure may temporarily fall to below pre-laugh levels, your muscles go limp, and you bask in a mellow euphoria." [7]

Many people are familiar with the story of Norman Cousins. He helped nurse himself back to health from a crippling condition by laughing, among other things. He was suffering from a disease of the connective tissue, that caused nodules to appear on his body, and made even moving difficult. When he was faced with the prognosis that there was no cure for his disease, he remembered having read the book, *The Stress of Life,* by Hans Selye.

Selye showed that adrenal exhaustion could be caused by emotional tension, such as frustration or suppressed rage, and detailed the negative effects of the negative emotions on body chemistry. Cousins reasoned that if negative emotions produce negative chemical changes in the body, wouldn't the positive emotions produce positive chemical changes. He thought, "Is it possible that love, hope, faith, laughter, confidence, and the will to live have therapeutic value? Do chemical changes occur only on the downside?" [8]

He talked with his doctor, who agreed to try this new approach, and after watching funny films and listening to books that made him laugh, he definitely started to heal. He went back to work at the *Saturday Review,* and eventually was well. He feels that his laughing, along with the injections of ascorbic acid (see chapter 7), positive faith, and healthy food, in addition to the support of his doctor and friends helped him recover from the disease that was destroying the body's connective tissue.

Notes

Introduction
1. Gayelord Hauser, *Gayelord Hauser's New Treasury of Secrets,* (New York, NY, Fawcett Crest, c. 1976), p. 24.

Chapter 1
1. Paul Lee Tan, ThD., *Encyclopedia of 7,700 Illustrations: Signs of the Times,* (Rockville, Maryland, Assurance Publishers, c.1988) p. 542.
2. Ibid., p. 775.
3. Ibid., pp. 775-776.

Chapter 3
1. Linda Clark, *Secrets of Health and Beauty,* (New York, NY, Jove Publications, c. 1969), p. 66.
2. Ibid., p. 69
3. Adelle Davis, *Let's Eat Right to Keep Fit,* (New York, NY, Harcourt Brace Jovanovich, Inc., c. 1970) pp. 131-132.
4. Earl Mindell, *Earl Mindell's Vitamin Bible,* (New York, NY, Warner Books, c.1985), p. 34.

Chapter 4
1. Earl Mindell, *Earl Mindell's Vitamin Bible,* (New York, NY, Warner Books, c.1985), p. 14.
2. Linda Clark, *Secrets of Health and Beauty,* (New York, NY, Jove Publications, c. 1969), p. 87.

Chapter 5
1. Linda Clark, *Secrets of Health & Beauty,* (New York, NY, Jove Publications, c. 1969).
2. Ibid., p. 56.
3. Gayelord Hauser, *Gayelord Hauser's New Treasure of Secrets,* (New York, Fawcett Crest Books, c. 1974) p. 23.
4. Ibid., p. 39.
5. Ibid., p. 39.
6. Ibid., p. 38.

Chapter 6

1. Gayelord Hauser, *Gayelord Hauser's New Treasury of Secrets,* (New York, NY, Fawcett Crest, c. 1974) p. 201.
2. Gayelord Hauser, *Look Youger-Live Longer*, (Farrar Straus & Co. N.Y. c. 1976).
3. Dr. Bruce B. Miller, *Nutrition for Beautiful Hair, Skin, and Nails,*(Dallas, TX, Bruce Miller Enterprises, Inc. c. 1993) p.8.
4. Ibid., p. 7.
5. Ibid., pp. 7-8.

Chapter 7

1. Walter Pierpaoli, M.D., PhD., and William Regelson, M.D., *The Melatonin Miracle, (*Simon & Schuster, New York, NY, c. 1995). p. 36.
2. Emmanuel Cheraskin: W. Marshall Ringsdorf: Emily Sisley, *The Vitamin C Connection* (Harper & Row, New York, NY, c. 1983), p. 185.
3. Norman Cousins, *Anatomy of an Illness as Perceived by the Patient,* (W.W. Norton & Co., c.1979), p.39-40.

Chapter 9

1. Adelle Davis, *Let's Eat Right to Keep Fit,* (New York, NY, Harcourt Brace Jovanovich, Inc. c. 1970). pp. 143, 165.
2. Ibid., pp. 150, 180.
3 Lesley Tierra, L.AC., Herbalist, *The Herbs of Life*, (The Crossing Press, CA, c. 1992), p. 157.
4. Walter Pierpaoli, M.D., Ph.D., and William Regelson, M.D., *The Melatonin Miracle*, p. 180.

Chapter 10

1. Bernie S. Siegel, M.D., *Love, Medicine & Miracles,* (Harper & Row Publishers, New York, NY, c. 1986), p. 68.
2. James F. Scheer, *Selenium Cancer Fighter,* Better Nutrition Magazine, June 1992, p.15.
3. Holly McCord, RD, *Nutrition News*, Prevention Magazine, April 1995, p. 54

4. Cheraskin, Ringsdorf, and Sisley, *The Vitamin C Connection*, p. 121.
5. Prevention Magazine, p. 52.
6. Earl Mindell, *Vitamin Bible,* (Werner Books, New York, NY, c. 1985), p. 15.

Chapter 12

1. Dr. Paavo Airola, *Juice Fasting*, (Sherwood, OR, Health Plus Publishers, c.1971), p. 22.
2. Ibid., p. 23.

Chapter 14

1. Siri Khalsa, *Nutrition News*, 1989 Vol. XII, No. 4 (Riverside, CA).

Chapter 16

1. Linda Clark, *Secrets of Health and Beauty*, p. 95.
2. Ibid., p. 105.
3. Ibid.
4. Ibid., p. 97.

Chapter 17

1. Gayelord Hauser, *Gayelord Hauser's New Treasury of Secrets*, (New York, NY, Fawcett Crest, c.1976), p. 161.

Chapter 18

1. Pierpaoli and Regelson, *The Melatonin Miracle,* p. 81.

Chapter 20

1. Pierpaoli and Regelson, *The Melatonin Miracle*, p. 108, 170-171.
2. Robert Ornstein, Ph.D. and David Sobel, M.D., *Healthy Pleasures*, (Addison-Wesley Publishing Company, Inc., Reading, Massachusetts, c.1989), p. 168.
3. Billie Jay Sahley, Ph.D. *The Anxiety Epidemic*, (San Antonia, TX, The Watercress Press, 1986).
4. Ornstein and Sobel, *Healthy Pleasures*, p. 60.

5. William Sadler, *Practice of Psychiatry* (St. Louis, C.V. Mosby Co., 1953), pp. 1012-1013.
6. Ornstein and Sobel, *Healthy Pleasures*, p. 221.
7. Ibid., p. 216.
8. Norman Cousins, *Anatomy of an Illness as Perceived by the Patient*, (W. W. Norton & Company, New York, NY, c1979), p. 35.

Epilogue
1. Eleanor King, *Guide to Glamor*, (Englewood Cliffs, N.J., Prentice-Hall, c. 1937).
2. Ibid.